What's Your
Magical Moment?

What's Your
Magical Moment?

Disconnect to Reconnect to Your Real Life

Beyond our hectic, fast-paced, demanding life,
there is a place and time where we can pause,
find meaning, get clarity, and experience joy.
I call these our magical moments…
Come, let me show you where.

By
Gina Kloes

NEW YORK

What's Your Magical Moment?
Disconnect to Reconnect to Your Real Life

Published in New York, New York, by Morgan James Publishing. Morgan James and The Entrepreneurial Publisher are trademarks of Morgan James, LLC. www.MorganJamesPublishing.com

The Morgan James Speakers Group can bring authors to your live event. For more information or to book an event visit The Morgan James Speakers Group at www.TheMorganJamesSpeakersGroup.com.

Morgan James Publishing
The Entrepreneurial Publisher
5 Penn Plaza, 23rd Floor, New York City, New York 10001
(212) 655-5470 office • (516) 908-4496 fax
www.MorganJamesPublishing.com

bitlit

A free eBook edition is available with the purchase of this print book.

CLEARLY PRINT YOUR NAME ABOVE IN UPPER CASE

Instructions to claim your free eBook edition:
1. Download the BitLit app for Android or iOS
2. Write your name in **UPPER CASE** on the line
3. Use the BitLit app to submit a photo
4. Download your eBook to any device

9781630474973   paperback
9781630474997   eBook

Library of Congress Control Number:
2015910410

Cover Design by:
3 Dog Design
www.3dogdesign.net
chris@3dogdesign.net

Interior Design by:
Brittany Bondar
www.Sage-Words.com

In an effort to support local communities, raise awareness and funds, Morgan James Publishing donates a percentage of all book sales for the life of each book to Habitat for Humanity Peninsula and Greater Williamsburg.

Get involved today, visit
www.MorganJamesBuilds.com

Habitat for Humanity®
Peninsula and
Greater Williamsburg
Building Partner

This book is dedicated to my five beautiful children

Justin, Oliver, and Samantha
The three children I brought into this world
and
Cristian and Ashton
The two children my amazing husband, Greg, brought into my life

In celebration of all of our magical moments together

Manhattan Beach, California
April 2015

ACKNOWLEDGEMENTS

There are so many people for whom I feel a true debt of gratitude for inspiring and supporting me in bringing my dream to reality in this book. There are so many more people than those listed below, and you know who you are and how you have touched my life. My inspiration and love continue to come from my family and friends and the magical moments we have shared over my lifetime.

Greg Kloes – My husband, the love of my life, my rock, and my best friend. You inspire me to live a life filled with integrity, blessings, courage, and strength. You give our family and me more than you ever expect to receive in return, and you are a gift to us all. I rely upon you as my guiding light, and you always help me find home. Thank you for all you do, and I thank God every day for the moment on 3-16 you came into my life.

Justin, Oliver, Sammy, Cristian, and Ashton – For all the magic and love we have shared over the years. You are what make my life worthwhile. You are an amazing group of children, and each of you has taught me many of the most important lessons in my life.

Oliver – You fill my heart with your kindness, tenacity, and focus to reach your dreams.

Sammy – You teach me to grow through your independence, spice, spirit, and love of life.

Cristian – You remind me of what is important through your intelligence, loyalty, and love.

Ashton – You lift my spirit with your creativity, sensitivity, and ability to experience the world through your amazing awareness.

Justin – You strengthen me through your perseverance through all odds.

I am thankful I can call each of you my child, and I love you more than words could ever describe. Thank you for creating some of the most magical moments in my life.

Justin Spizman – You literally brought tears to my eyes with your work. It was an amazing journey together, and I am thankful for your edits and feedback. You helped me bring a beautiful story to life and share magical moments with the world. Without you, the magic would have just remained in my mind.

Scott Frishman – Thank you for gently guiding me and inspiring me to complete this dream and share these magical moments. I am so appreciative to have learned more about your family and the magical moments you have shared over the years. This book wouldn't have come to life without you. Author101 paved the way and you gave my journey new light, care and wisdom.

Melissa – Thank you for supporting me as this book became a reality. You lifted me at times I could not lift myself and are constantly by my side to celebrate life's victories. This book is as much for you as it is because of you.

Woody – You are one of those friends who remind me and so many others to find the joy in our lives when we can't see it ourselves. You have kept me laughing at times I wanted to cry and made me belly-laugh until I couldn't breathe! Our hysterical and soul friendship is meaningful beyond words.

The Anthony Robbins Trainers For Good – Thanks goes to my chosen family. I am honored and blessed to belong to a group of over one hundred extraordinary people from all over the world who continue to do good in this world while holding each other to exceptionally high standards in all areas of life. We are there for each other in a heartbeat, and many of the people in this family have cheered me on to complete this project. Thank you for always being by my side and helping to change the world.

Kellie Lancaster – You are the scaffolding that holds our business and our life together. I could not wish or hope for a more dedicated and professional team.

Dr. Ruth Newton – Thank you for the wisdom, grace, and love you give to all those you serve. Light and the gifts from the universe come in so many forms, and you are an angel in this world and an inspiration now and always.

The contributors – Thank you to all the people who contributed their personal magical moments to this book. You have given me a sacred trust with the special memories from your life. I will hold these moments in light and love. I am hopeful I did each one of your stories justice and honored your family, friends, and you.

Anthony Robbins – Thank you for your insights and teachings that have inspired me to take charge of my life, create my own destiny, and live the life of my dreams.

Deepak Chopra, MD, and David Simon, MD – Thank you for your wisdom and helping me find love, light, healing, and inspiration in my body, mind, spirit, and beyond. Dr. Chopra, you swirl the heavens; Dr. Simon, you bring heaven to earth. As one of your students and one of your Chopra Center University teachers, I am ever grateful.

Snatam Kaur – Your music is a guiding light to my heart and the magical moments that bring my life meaning. Your gifts inspire and awaken the spirit in this world.

George Frye – A special heartfelt and warm thank-you to my father, who passed away in 1985. Although you are gone, the magical moments and love you gave to me during your life are enough to fill many lifetimes.

CONTENTS

7   The Magic of Time Alone   139

8   The Magical Gifts in Nature   161

Dear Reader,

I originally started writing this book because some of my friends dared me to do so. Together, we agreed to individually create a book on a subject about which we were passionate.

I have always loved friendly competition, and this moment was no different. I immediately began to consider the topic. My answer quickly appeared. Experiencing, appreciating, and sharing magical moments has always been a profound part of my life. Just ask my kids. We share magical moments at our family meals, celebrations, and especially when we are with friends. Big and small, these magical moments have been integral parts of our lives. Over the years, I discovered you learn a lot about someone by listening to their personal stories – their own magical moments. It is an honor and privilege I don't take lightly.

As the days turned into months, our deadline for the completion of our competition quickly approached. Deborah Battersby and Michelle Scarafile finished their books. While I was happy for their success, it was clear my mindset shifted from winning the competition to creating a valuable message from my heart and soul. It became more about doing it right rather than just doing it. I wanted this book to be a reflection of the importance of remembering our stories, finding the magic in those stories, and then sharing them with others. Because let's be honest – the best part of any story is sharing it with others. As I dove deeper into this project and listened to the magical moments from others, I was happy to let the deadline pass and celebrate Deborah and Michelle claiming their prizes. My prize is the work in this book.

I am hopeful you will share in my experience. When reading this book, I also hope you set an intention to locate these moments. This is a book about stories from our lives. Within those stories are magical moments that shape who we are in this world. To get the most out of this book, you have to reflect on your potential outcomes for reading it. Are you here to discover the meaning of magical moments? Do you have a life-time of memories and would like an easy way to capture the magic in those moments to share with your loved ones? Are you seeking to experience more magical moments in your own life and the lives of those around you? Are you looking for the magic in your life? Do you just want some time to enjoy magical moments written by others? You may want all of these. Set your intention for reading this book, and enjoy the process.

Within these pages you will find my personal definition of magical moments. You will find moments written by many people who have found the magic in their own lives. Some of those moments will resonate with you. Through the joy, the laughter, the sorrow, the pain, and the reflection in all of the stories you will read, people found the magic and meaning in those moments. They discovered what was truly meaningful and life changing in each experience. And so can you.

This journey was always a very personal one to me. I was often told by friends and loved ones that I have a way of inspiring them to create "magical moments." The more I thought about it, the more I realized that I might actually have a gift for helping those around me to find unbelievably special and cherished opportunities. I strive to help people find the most nourishing and enlivening meaning within their life experiences. This book is a culmination of those skills and desire and my hope is that my guidance will help you to disconnect from something so you can reconnect to everything.

Together, we will journey down the path of creating "magical moments." As with everyone interviewed and featured in this book, my goal is to connect with you and your story so I can play a small role in elevating the quality of the moments you live. I did it with people with whom I connected to write this book, and I am confident I can also do it with you. Our paths are intersecting for a reason and my continued hope is that together we can enjoy the process of capturing life's true gems.

This book is your guide to find the magic outside of these pages and within your own life. To help you, throughout the book are sections offering you the opportunity to pause and reflect on aspects of your own life. You will have the chance to discover how those moments shaped who you are in this world. It's possible that you have yet to uncover the magic and find the gifts from those experiences. Now is the time to discover and appreciate each of those moments before they are overlooked forever.

Shifting your perspective to finding the magic in life's moments may not occur overnight. Allow yourself to enjoy the process and take the time you need to look and discover the magical moments in your life. Periodically disconnect from your modern life and set aside a little bit of time to find the magic in your life. Most importantly, pause to experience, reflect, and savor all the magical moments as they occur around you and to you each and every day.

In celebration of the magic in all of our lives, enjoy this book.

With magic and love,

Gina Kloes

1

Getting Lost in the Shuffle

Live with intention. Walk to the edge.
Listen hard. Practice wellness. Play with abandon. Laugh.
Choose with no regret. Appreciate your friends.
Continue to learn. Do what you love.
Live as if this is all there is.

– Mary Anne Radmacher

Well-respected polymath, astronomer, physician, philosopher, and poet Omar Khayyam advises, "Be happy for this moment, this moment is your life…."

If you wanted to learn to cook, you could attend a cooking class. What about becoming a doctor? Medical school, right? Or even a lawyer? I would bet law school might be on your mind. But what if you wanted to live life to its fullest and build an amazingly meaningful and purpose-driven life? You know, one that is grounded in the celebration of exciting moments on a daily basis. Life offers us great opportunities to smile, allows our hearts to sing, and projects the warmth we feel in our souls. The education of life comes through the moments encompassing our lives.

There is no class, school, or education program to build the perfect life. But there is no doubt in my mind that any great life consists of taking the enormous amount of magical moments and celebrating them in a thoughtful and appreciative manner. Life is filled with time, and time is filled with moments. These moments are like beautiful snowflakes falling from the sky, each one unique and exceptional. Every moment both valued and respected achieves a wonderful celebration of time. Time moves fast and can be lost. But it can also be celebrated, and this book will help you accomplish just that. But before we dive into how to create and cherish these moments, let's take time to reflect and evaluate on our lives to determine what may be hindering our ability to truly stop and smell the roses.

Our Hectic, Fast-Paced, Demanding Lives

We live in a hectic and fast-paced world. Some days we barely have time to catch our breath, let alone take a moment to appreciate or even notice the exceptional moments in our lives. In modern society, we are over stimulated and overworked. A recent study of twenty-five hundred American workers conducted by CareerBuilder.com found that 77 percent feel burned-out at their jobs. The truth is many of us long for something more meaningful. The challenge is that we have difficulty finding time, even just a moment, to discover what that means individually.

Time passes – days into months, months into years, years into decades, and decades into a lifetime. The moments of our lives tend to be lost in a whirlwind of daily routines, to-do lists, and jam-packed schedules. Our spirits are left empty because our minds are constantly distracted. We are too busy to appreciate and acknowledge the magic and special moments in our lives *while* they happen because we are constantly focused on the *next* task.

At the end of our lives, too many of us reflect back and regret the times we let the special moments go uncelebrated and unappreciated.

Starting right now, your life can be different. Beyond our hectic, fast-paced, demanding world, there is a place and time where we can pause, find meaning, get clarity, experience joy, and reconnect to your real life. I call these our magical moments.

There is magic in all of our experiences. It is in those moments that we receive the lessons, growth, and gifts that fulfill our lives. Sometimes we don't always appreciate the significance of a moment until after it happens. If we pause to truly *experience* those moments while they are happening, we can fully realize that with both the joys and challenges in life there is a message, a gift, and a lesson to be learned. Whether we know it or not, the meanings we give those magical moments shape our lives.

Come; let me show you where to find them.

REFLECT

- When was the last time you took a moment to pause and find meaning in your life?

- Recall a very special moment in your life; what lessons did you learn in that moment?
- Recall the last time you shared a joyful moment with someone you love—your child, your parent, a significant other...
- When was the last time you felt complete peace and calm?
- When was the last time you felt truly loved?
- When was the last time you felt truly happy?
- How do you appreciate your life experiences and the way they shaped who you are today?

Earn More, Do More, Have More

We move at 100 miles per minute. Sadly, there is a common notion that our true value is directly related to how much we earn or how many things we own. Modern society is plagued by the constant need and pressure to earn more, do more, and have more. Unfortunately, these expectations eventually lead us to resentment and a feeling of overwhelming disappointment. This leaks into our lives and can impact our mind and body, influencing our coworkers, our family, our home, and our entire environment and lifestyle.

We feel it and then teach our children to do the same. It is a difficult cycle to break. Children learn they must work harder and achieve more to have more in life. In a recent article published on healthychildren.org ("When the Pressure to Excel Gets Out of Hand"), Dr. William Lord Coleman of Duke University Medical Center and the University of North Carolina School of Medicine explains that pressure on our children is a national phenomenon with two distinct causes. First, in an increasingly high-tech economy, there are more demands on tomorrow's high-tech workers. Second, more and more parents get "revved" up about their children needing to do well in school so they can get into good colleges. "Some of their concerns are justified," [Dr. Coleman] continues, "but other times they're focused too far ahead and not on keeping their youngster's life balanced now."

Despite their best intentions, many parents who genuinely care about their children become models of stress and conflict. Children learn and practice what they experience in life, and there are very few role models for joy, peace, and calm.

People are role models in life not by what they say but rather by who they are as people and how they live their lives every day. Children especially model the lives their parents lead. One of the most profound references a child has about how to live a life comes from their families. Although society, the media, and peers provide other references to life, children experience life with their families every day. What they see, hear, and feel through their families is a powerful part of their beliefs and experiences in life.

Think about what you learned from your childhood and family. Were they shining examples of how to live a fulfilling life, or were they glaring warnings of what not to do? The notions of "have more" and "do more" are infectious. But they do not have to be. You have the power to break the cycle, sever the chain, and rework your life so it is not grounded in earn more, do more, have more, but rather in live more, breathe more, and find more magical moments.

REFLECT

- What are some of the experiences you remember from your childhood?
- What are some of the lessons and gifts you learned from those memories?
- How can you find gratitude for those moments, even the most challenging ones, knowing how your life is today?

Online and Disconnected

Without a doubt, we find a direct correlation between who we are and how we were raised. The seeds of success or failure are planted at an early age. As we mature and grow older, we become more dedicated to our habits and behaviors, good or bad. Shifting to a life based on the beautiful moments and not the tangible things is the first step to securing a euphoric happiness. The environment of our lives is one distinctly different from that of our parents and older generations – meaning we may be a product of those who raised us, but we are also a result of the atmosphere in which we live.

Today we run through our lives in an extremely fast-paced manner. The only way to keep up is to rely heavily on the technology that keeps us connected. But as we exchange face-to-face communication for screen-to-screen connections, we are becoming increasingly less connected. Magical moments are created in real life by touch, sight, sounds, smell, and experiencing those moments firsthand. If you are not present, the gifts are not the same. With that in mind, we need to disconnect our disconnection and grow into individuals who are literally present for the presents life offers.

Consider the following magical moment of a family who realized they had strayed from their purpose and decided to reconnect:

Up in Smoke – *A Family Disconnected*

> *I arrived home from work to a cursory nod from my son, as his eyes remained glued to his new video game. I asked him to turn down the volume. I don't think he heard me. I shouted up to my daughter to set the table. She replied, "Five more minutes while I upload these photos to Facebook." My husband finally arrived home from a typical long day still on a conference call and signaled to me that he was heading up to his office to finish his emails.*

While I was making dinner, I was distracted by the all too familiar sound of an incoming text message. As usual, I was drawn to look at the message and respond. It seems that not replying to people immediately has become this century's new mortal sin. One text message led to a twenty-minute video chat on my new iPhone with one of my friends.

During my video chat, my friend looked concerned and asked me what the smoke was behind me. As I turned around, I realized the dinner I had started was up in smoke. I realized with all of us completely immersed in our own technological worlds, no one noticed the smoke clouds slowly developing in the kitchen. But it was too late. The smoke triggered the most unbearable sound: the screeching of our very effective and very annoying fire alarms.

The whole family frantically arrived in the kitchen opening the windows and even fanning the smoke with iPads and anything else to make it stop. We all turned as my daughter started snapping photos on her cell phone. "What are you looking at? I need to post these on Facebook. I have to take a picture or it didn't happen."

As the smoke died down, we all burst into belly laughs realizing the absurdity of the whole situation. It was in that moment that I recognized it had been a long time since we laughed as a family or even did something together. The alarm did much more than alert me that I had ruined my beautiful tri-tip dinner. I realized we needed a way to disconnect from online worlds so that we could reconnect with each other.

It is inevitable that we are now and forever affected by technology. The exponential technological advances have profoundly impacted our lives in both positive and negative ways. They have reduced a once rich and flourishing environment to one where magical moments could be few and far in between. The manner in which we communicate simply does not lead to opportunities to connect. Texts, emails, cell phones, and the Internet have replaced face-to-face communications. Information now moves at unimaginable speeds, but keeping up with the speed of information can be overwhelming.

Communication is essential to life. It is as important as the water we drink or the air we breathe. We have no connectivity without it. Communication through modern technology allows us to virtually connect with an endless number of people. With the click of a single keystroke, we can send messages simultaneously to friends around the world, even friends we have never met in person but have "friended" online. With another click, we can post messages that reach millions. We can have friends in online communities, buy food and clothing through online shopping sites, obtain college degrees through virtual universities, pay bills online, and hold videoconferences for work meetings. Despite these many advantages, this virtual world challenges one significant part of our lives: our real world. Most of us are so connected online, rather than with one another, that we completely miss the chance to experience the magical real-life moments in our lives.

In order to live more meaningful lives amidst an overwhelming influx of technological devices, we should seek ways to use technology instead of allowing technology to use us. There was a time when we had relationships with people rather than machines. We used to connect with people in person, through real live phone calls and simple one-on-one conversations over coffee. We understood when someone was actually irritated by his or her tone, inflection, and body language rather than rereading an email or text attempting to interpret the writer's intent. Today we replace a lunch date with checking a newsfeed; we nearly walk into traffic while texting; we take hundreds of pictures to post instead of just pausing to experience a moment of real time.

Who Rescued Whom? – *A Tale of Two Brothers*

My little brother worries me. Wait, correction, he scares me.

I'm seven years older but I feel like we are worlds apart. I'm out-going and enjoy making new friends. Kody is the opposite. I've seen his transformation from a once smiley kid to an isolated loner. He no longer has to go out of his comfort zone for enter-tainment or activities after school. Kody just plops down in front of the computer claiming to do homework or zones out in video games. Don't get me wrong, I love my Xbox too, but it's like his girlfriend. At this rate, he will probably never have one. I'm sur-prised his eyeballs haven't burned out from staring at his laptop screen for so long.

Oh, and forget about making eye contact with him. His awkward-ness seems contagious. When he is around even I start to feel awkward. "Hey, man, what's new with you?" And, as usual, he has nothing to say. Crickets. I took it personally for a while, but then I just gave up even trying.

The other week I was at home visiting from college. Out of pure, selfish boredom I asked Kody to hang out.

"Let's go do something," I said. "I'll even pay."

"It's raining," he mumbled over his Xbox controller.

"Let's go bowling, or anything. Dude, you are never going to make any new friends. You don't do anything," I insisted.

"That's boring. I'm busy," said Kody. Conversation over.

He continued in his zombie-like state for the rest of the weekend. I gave up and went to hang out with friends.

I was still at home one afternoon when Kody came home from school. It was ice cold outside, the kind of cold that chills you to your bones. I heard him kick off his boots and dart right up to his room, nothing out of the ordinary for him. Moments had passed, and then I heard strange noises coming from his room. I went up to investigate.

As the door creaked open, I was shocked to find a litter of puppies running around his room, wreaking havoc, whining, and looking very scared. One even left a little present in the corner.

"You have to help!" Kody shouted. "Mom is going to kill me, but I found them in a box in an alley on the walk home. I couldn't...I couldn't just leave them there. Who would leave them there? It's freezing!" He was a little choked up and was chaotically trying to corral them together.

I really wanted to say no way. I was a little surprised by this whole situation. I didn't want to spend the rest of my college break play-ing the part of the ASPCA, but there was something about the look in his eyes that told me I was going to be in "puppy land" for a while. I canceled most of my plans with old friends, and we spent the whole next week trying to find homes for the puppies.

The shelter was not an option as the puppies could end up being euthanized. Kody was determined to find them good homes. To make that happen, he was finally forced to step out of his safe little world of electronic toys. Hah! Welcome to the real world, buddy!

In truth, we had so much fun with the little fur balls that it finally gave us something to talk about. We walked around the neighbor-hood putting up posters; we went door to door asking neighbors, friends, and family for good homes. I posted an ad online, and we had a couple of people from Craigslist stop by. My brother grilled them to make sure they would provide suitable, loving homes. I was proud to be a part of this experience with him. He was meet-ing new people, talking to strangers – and, boy, did he love those puppies.

By the time I had to head back to college, we only had one pup left. He was the runt of the litter and was a little skittish. My brother seemed particularly attached to this dog. Kody let him sleep with him at night. The dog never left his side. There was a spark back in Kody's life. I was so used to his lifeless video eyes that I forgot what it was like to see him really happy. He finally felt truly connected to something alive instead of just to his computer and video games. Luckily, my parents agreed to let him keep the dog.

"I think I like the name Cooper. Cooper my alley dog!" he said. You could see the excitement in his eyes.

I come home to visit once a month and have been watching my brother's transformation. Slowly, but surely, the days that he was glued to the Xbox or computer have become a thing of the past. Instead he walks Cooper or plays with him in the park. I even noticed he met a few kids from the neighborhood on those walks, and they started coming over to the house. Kody doesn't scare me anymore. What scares me is that I almost missed that chance, that moment, to help him rediscover a connection to a real life. But I didn't miss it. I decided to help him rescue the puppies that day. Sometimes I still wonder...who really rescued who?

Our children are exceptionally vulnerable to the effects of our digital life. Instead of learning the important art of personal interaction, many children grow up socially awkward and find their safety and comfort in a security blanket made up of computers, cell phones, and video games. Remember, the apple doesn't fall far from the tree. Are we really will-ing to raise a generation of children whose best memories are online virtual experiences, or are we willing ourselves to disconnect and take the time to create real-life magical moments and experiences?

REFLECT

- Consider ways to find more real-life magical moments in your life by turning off technology.
- What other positive ways could you find to experience real life with the people you love?
- How much time do you spend each day with your family disconnected from technology?
- When was the last time you had an in-person, one-on-one meaningful chat with a close friend?
- What would have to happen for you to take a moment each day to pause and really be present with someone?

Positions, Possessions, and Power

An exciting transformation will happen once we begin the shift from cellular communication to personal communication. Focusing on people and not the convenience of communication is the first step in manifesting the opportunity for more magical moments. Adjusting our own attitudes can increase the chance for moments that have enormous meaning. Many of us are defined by what we do, what we have, and what we control. If you ask someone who they are, they usually will respond with a description of their roles in life, the things they own, or the influence they have with others. "I am a mother. I am a teacher. I am an expert in social media. I am a homeowner. I am a Mac user. I run a multinational corporation."

Beyond our positions, possessions, and power, we are so much more. We are the mathematical equivalent of our magical moments. That is what truly defines our lives. At times we can all crave something in life beyond being a servant to our roles and the things we own – yet many of us are at a loss on how to start that journey of discovery. If we don't have clarity about our identity, we are at the mercy of other people's definitions and leave our future and our life in their hands. So let's take some time to evaluate how we view our positions, our possessions, and our relationships with power and control.

Positions

We play so many roles in the course of our lifetimes. We are parents, daughters, sons, spouses, employees, and members of a modern society, among others. Each of our roles creates expectations, pressure, and commitments for our lives. Dr. Humphry Osmond, an expert on the roles people play in life, explains: "Socially defined roles are difficult to change because each one of them confers rights upon, and exacts obligations from, those who play them."

Who Am I? Who Am I Really? – *A Woman's Journey to Find Her Life*

My father was a good man and lived his life believing he was doing good for his children. He taught me that to live a good life, I needed to first be a good wife. Second, I needed to be a good mother and to raise my children to grow up to be self-sufficient, healthy, and successful so I could be a proud mother. Lastly, he said, "Work hard so you will be a success in business." As I grew older, I set my targets to accomplish all three of these things. I married the man I loved and was a devoted wife. We had a son and I became a devoted mother. I worked very hard and became the successful entrepreneur my father always envisioned for me. Life was just as I planned.

Then, as happens with many people, my marriage fell apart and I went through a painful divorce. Suddenly I was single and not the "wife" my father imagined for me. My son left for college and started his own life. In 2008, the financial crisis hit our economy and the business I helped start fell apart. I felt like I had nothing left of value with me. All that I had hoped to become and my father dreamed for me was gone. Now what?

I felt purposeless; I felt lost. I sought meaning for my life and clarity on what to do next. Why was I on this earth?

Many people I knew who had similar challenges turned to alcohol, some to drugs. Prescription medications and other drugs seemed so readily available for them. I didn't want that for my life. I had already seen the destructive effects drug abuse can have on so many lives. Although I felt intense sadness and grief, I knew there was more.

A friend asked me what I liked to do. I frankly had absolutely no idea. My life had been so structured, busy, and planned. Now the world and all the possibilities seemed so overwhelming. For days I just stayed within the safety of my home not feeling ready to venture out for anything. Eventually that became old and I knew it was time for something else.

I actually browsed the bookstore and found several books that piqued my interest. I loved the mountains and often dreamed about exploring nature from the vista of a great mountain peak. I called a few friends I hadn't seen in years. Before, I never had time to really see anyone other than my employees and my family. I started going on long walks listening to new music and discovering how great it felt to finally get some exercise. I began brainstorming new business ideas for things I would never have considered before. I had always followed the lead set by my father and never thought to stray for even a moment. I realized that life had so much more to offer me than the three roles that had dominated my life for so long.

The magic in losing all the structured positions in my life – wife, mother, and successful entrepreneur – was that now I could explore who I was and what would really make me happy. I learned that our lives couldn't be defined by any particular roles we play. Those many roles in our lives have a beginning, middle, and an end, yet life goes on. I am now willing to try most anything and have one primary rule: if I like it, I'll probably do it again. If I don't, I won't! My life now is defined by my constant and never-ending journey of discovery, a role I don't anticipate ending any-time soon.

Why do we define so much of our value by the title we have before or after our name? It is one part nature, another part nurture, and an unhealthy reliance on the need for acceptance. When you welcome magical moments in your life, you begin to reorganize how you value segments of your life. Titles mean less; moments of happiness with friends and family mean more. Developing an awareness of our magical moments allows us to have a childlike sense of wonder and truly discover the exciting parts of life that were once lost.

In the course of a day, we constantly switch roles and do our best to meet changing demands. In the midst of all these transitions, there is little to encourage us to take a moment to breathe in and appreciate the moments as we live them. Those moments are our foundation and make up the story of our lives. Even more importantly, there is magic in many of these moments that can give meaning, clarity, and joy to our lives if we don't miss them as we focus on playing role after role.

REFLECT

- How do you define yourself?
- How does this definition impact your life?
- Who are you really in this world?

Possessions

Modern society teaches us that we should work harder simply to obtain more "things." However, those newly acquired possessions also come with more responsibilities and time commitments. Whether it's a house, a car, a computer, a new outfit, or even the latest greatest new gadget, it requires not only money to buy it but also space to keep it, time to clean it, resources to maintain it, insurance to protect it, and even more money and time for its upkeep in the future. In our overzealousness to have more, along with everything else we have acquired, we often lose the time to really enjoy those things. Do we even take time to question whether all the effort to acquire something was actually worth it? Did that *something* give real meaning and joy to our lives?

What Makes You Happy – *A Story of a New Life*

> *Sitting in our new home, reflecting back over the last few years, I am ever grateful for one magical question that changed my perspective on how to create a home filled with happiness and treasured memories.*

> *It was a sunny San Diego day, and I walked through the house putting things in piles preparing to move to a new home with my fiancé. There were supposed to be three piles: one pile of things to donate, one pile to throw out, and one to move to our new house. I toured each room, rummaging through various things I had accumulated over the years, and had a conversation with myself that went something like this:*

>> *"I need to keep these things; they were so expensive!"*
>> *"My children grew up with these things. They will need these things to feel like home."*
>> *"I have had all of these things forever. I couldn't part with them now."*

"This was my mother's; she would be so upset if I didn't take it with me."
"This was a gift from my best friend in high school. Wow, those were the days."

By the time I went through all the bedrooms and the living room, there was only one pile in each room—everything was coming with me! When my fiancé, Greg, arrived at the house to check my progress, he looked around and said, "What is this?"

I responded, "These are all the things I'm taking. There is this guitar I have had since I was a teen. Someday I will play it again. My mom gave me this black lacquered cabinet from Chinatown. I'm sure we'll find a place for it. I bought those overalls many years ago, and I'm sure I will fit in them again sometime soon. This red leather jacket was SO expensive. I'm not sure I have ever worn it, but I just can't give it away. I guess I'm bringing everything. We can always rent a storage unit if we can't find room in our new house."

In the kindest and gentlest tone he could muster, Greg replied, "We are starting again."

We walked back to the first bedroom and he looked at me and said, "We have a new system. For each item in this house, I want you to ask 'does this make me happy and I mean REALLY HAPPY?' If it does, it comes with us; if it doesn't, out it goes!"

Room after room we went. I quickly realized that there were very few things I owned that really made me happy. In fact, I found one of the few things I treasured that made me feel true joy buried in the bottom of a box in the back of a closet. It was my father's two-tone dancing shoe. His life had such meaning because of the joy and passion he had for ballroom dancing. That shoe was definitely coming! Throughout the house we went on collecting trea-

sures and eliminating clutter. It was freeing, and I was now very excited about creating our new home.

Magic happened that one afternoon. I am now surrounded by joy. As time passed, I started asking that question about more than just things. Who in my life really makes me happy? What activities do I routinely do that really make me happy? I started clearing through that clutter too. Looking back, it all started with a simple magical question asked by a loving and wise man on a warm San Diego afternoon walking through rooms filled with my past and paving the way to my new happy home with my children and the man I love.

By taking inventory of your "things," you can indirectly take an even more important inventory of your life. By recognizing and evaluating what you don't need, you will better position yourself to identify what you do need and what really makes you happy. Magic happens when you decide to exchange tangible items for magical moments. In the long run, one will leave you feeling empty, the other completely fulfilled. You will never have "buyer's remorse" after investing time in those you love and care for deeply. Magical moments do not break down, they don't require constant upkeep, and they certainly don't require monthly payments.

REFLECT

- What things in your life truly make you happy?
- What things could you throw out?
- What would it mean for your life to open up some space for new possibilities?

Power

In Deepak Chopra's book *The Seven Spiritual Laws of Success*, he teaches, "When you seek power and control over other people, you waste energy. When you seek power for the sake of the ego, you spend energy chasing the illusion of happiness instead of enjoying happiness in the moment."

Oftentimes we define our success by the amount of influence we have on others. This could mean we are the boss, the head of a household, the coach of a team, the principal of a school, or anyone in a so-called "leadership role." Far too often people use power and control for the purpose of the addictive-like fulfillment it provides. Power, in this way, not only corrupts but also injects poison into relationships. Meaningful relationships are built on mutual respect and admiration, not on titles and job descriptions.

That's not to say that influencing others should be viewed as a negative behavior. In fact, some of the greatest leaders in our world lead by their genuine personalities, their integrity, and their authentic care for this world. Most magical moments occur when one person makes a difference in the life of another. But influence should come from a place of generosity, love, and vision, not self-fulfillment and greed. Only when influence is motivated by positive factors can true harmony be reached and magic can happen.

REFLECT

- Whom do you most admire in life?
- Who has had the most influence in your life?
- Who do you believe are the greatest leaders in our world?
- What qualities about them most inspire you?

The Epidemic of Depression, Anxiety, and Frustration

Positions, possessions, and power can create unwanted and unnecessary boundaries in your life. They limit your ability to find and achieve an enlightening place of happiness. When you allow your life to be fueled or driven by these 3 P's, you can eventually break down. The inevitable result will not be happiness but can be a dark world filled with depression, anxiety, and frustration.

Depression, anxiety, and frustration plague our society. More and more children and adults are afflicted with these serious conditions and continue to suffer. Various therapies are used to try to help people rise above these challenges, and yet the statistics increase.

The National Center for Health Statistics indicates that between 2005 and 2008, antidepressants were the third most common prescription drug taken by Americans of all ages and were most frequently used by persons aged eighteen to forty-four. That same study found even more disturbing news. From approximately 1988 to 2008, the rate of antidepressant use in the United States increased 400 percent among all ages. The report also found that females are two and a half times as likely to take antidepressant medication as males, concluding that 23 percent of women aged forty to fifty-nine take antidepressants, which is more than in any other age-sex group.

Mental health problems accounted for 156 million visits to doctors' offices, clinics, and hospital outpatient departments in 2005. Furthermore, the National Institute of Mental Health (NIMH) found that one in four women would experience severe depression at one point in their life.

These statistics are startling considering that much of the focus in treating depression and other mental illness has historically concentrated on medication and psychotherapy aimed at relieving symptoms. In our tendency to get caught up in our fast-paced lives, we look for a quick fix or the latest fast-acting relief rather than discovering the root cause.

As Martin E. P. Seligman, PhD, states in his book *Authentic Happiness*, "People who are impoverished, depressed, or suicidal care about much more than just the relief of their suffering. These persons care – sometimes desperately – about virtue, about purpose, about integrity and about meaning. Experiences that induce positive emotions cause negative emotions to dissipate rapidly."

Only when we identify the cause of unhappiness can we begin to treat it. Depression is an epidemic and medication is not the cure. It is simply a Band-Aid that only temporarily hides the pain. However, once you stop medicating, the pain quickly returns. The ultimate goal is to develop coping mechanisms to reduce your depression and shift your life to be grounded in happiness and exciting, meaningful moments. As we move through the next chapter of this book, you will find solutions to the epidemic of an unhappy life. Together we will begin the transformation, the shift, to a fulfilling life where magical moments are the rule, not the exception. If we are motivated and inspired to change our vantage point, there is a genuine happiness we can all achieve that will better our lives and the world as a whole.

REFLECT

- Have you ever felt depressed?
- If you could create a life of your dreams, what would that be?
- How would that life make you feel?
- Can you remember a time when you felt those feelings?
- Go back to that time now. What did you see? What did you hear? What were the specific feelings you felt at that time?
- What is one thing you could do right now to feel those feelings again?

2

Reconnecting to a Fulfilling and Happy Life

We don't remember days, we remember moments.

– Author Unknown

The Stories of Our Lives

It has been said that sometimes you don't realize the value of a moment until it becomes a memory. A life with purpose is truly an amazing prospect. And it is one that we can reach. People seek a way to be happy, peaceful, and calm in a world full of chaos and challenge. We all want to live with meaning, clarity, fulfillment, and happiness. Sometimes we cannot locate these things in our rush to meet the expectations of our hectic day-to-day lives. Our lives are simply muddied by all the moving pieces that we allow to divert our attention away from the meaningful moments. Happiness is not something that can be bought, found online, or owned. In fact, the more you attempt to "commodify" it, the less of a chance you will have to achieve it. But it doesn't have to be that way.

Whether my kids realized it or not, while they were growing up we were sharing magical moments. In my mind, I would take note of those times and appreciate our magic together, knowing there would come a day when they would no longer be children. I would always be their mom, but someday they would be adults with families of their own. I was determined to share time with them when I could still tuck them in at night, kiss them on their head, listen to their dating stories as teens, and watch them grow.

You can learn so much about other people by asking them what is magical in their life and listening to their magical moments. You may sometimes be surprised to hear what others believe is magical. In those moments you discover what people hold as important, what they value in life, and what is most memorable to them.

I have found that this is especially true with our children. When we share magical moments at our dinner table, I learn so much about my children and how their lives are developing.

Sometimes we get so caught up in our own beliefs and rules about life that it is helpful to remember that other people don't hold the same to be true. One of the most important "rules of the game" is that when someone shares a magical moment, you must not judge them. Anthony Robbins, Peak Performance strategist and a world authority on leadership psychology, teaches,"the moment you judge someone, you lose all ability to influence him or her." When you judge someone it really says more about your own beliefs and rules in life, making you less open to learning about the life of someone else.

In our attempts to love and teach our children, we as parents often want to correct, direct, and shape their lives. Sharing magical moments is not the time to do this. The moment you start judging someone's magical moment, especially if you do it openly, they can, and often will, shut down.

"People don't care how much you know until they know how much you care" is one of the most profound teachings of John C. Maxwell, an internationally recognized leadership expert. Consider your time spent sharing magical moments with loved ones as a sacred trust. Care about them, respect their magic, and appreciate that we all are unique in this world. Be open, be curious, be grateful that people, including your children, will open up and share their life stories with you.

So how can we create a life and still experience these things?

Surprise – *Gina's Story*

> *Driving home from work, I was tired and weary. The last thing I wanted to do was go out to dinner with friends. I had another extremely busy week ahead with business meetings out of town, piles of work at the office, and the kids' schedules to organize. Tomorrow there was more work and a long list of basketball games, cheerleading events, homework, and household chores. There was no end in sight for the rest of the week's activities. I*

could only dream of a nice cup of tea, a warm blanket, and my journal. It had been weeks, or was it months, since I had opened that book. As I walked in the front door, my husband's warm smile and embrace lifted my spirits.

Off we went to dinner amid my litany of complaints, "I'm too tired. I don't want to go!" We finally arrived at our friend's house, and as I walked in the front door, the cheering and music stopped me in my tracks.

"Why are Carolyn, Melissa, Nick, and all my other friends here?" I asked my husband. Then it hit me. This party was for me...celebrating my fiftieth birthday. As I grasped the reality of the evening, I scanned the room and a flood of magical moments swept me down memory lane. These people were from all different times and parts of my life. We all shared so much together—fifty years of joy, tears, laughter, sorrow, and so much more.

- *Belly laughing with Carolyn after too many long nights of work.*
- *My first kiss from my loving husband, looking into his tender eyes and knowing he was my true love.*
- *Bringing in the New Year surfing (at least trying to surf) at sunset with Tad. How silly we were to think the tourists were photographing us and not the breathtaking sunset behind us...the scent of the fresh ocean air still carries me right back onto my freshly waxed surfboard.*
- *Crying over my son's illness while baking cinnamon rolls with Patti. I can still taste the freshly baked icing sprinkled with my salty tears.*
- *Sacred, quiet moments with Kelly seeking guidance and support. Hearing her thoughtful words and prayers, and feeling her genuine concern and care.*

- *Dawnie and Dave, wow, there was a season of my life when I actually had time to have fun trying to learn to play volleyball at the beach – seems like an eternity ago.*
- *After we moved to Manhattan Beach, feeling such gratitude and appreciation for Nick as he guided and supported my son Oliver to earn his place and be accepted by the players at our local gym's pickup basketball games.*
- *Helping my friend Melissa move her oldest daughter into her college dorm for the first day of college...a tear in one eye, a smile in the other.*
- *And a lifetime of other magical moments.*

As I paused with gratitude and love, I remembered the moments of my life as they came to me one by one, like a touching movie of five decades, each with its own emotions, people, places, and lessons. For a brief moment, I relived them all with the sights, sounds, and feelings all held in my memory...the magical moments that have created my life.

I am now fifty-two, and it was only a fleeting moment ago that I was twenty-one. There has been a lot of life in my years. Some of those moments feel as if they were yesterday, while many are now only distant memories. Reflecting back fifty years, could I remember something magical and special about each year? How about each decade? What would my life be like if I had captured those memories and the gifts in each experience? What if I were able to leave those magical moments as a legacy to my children and my grandchildren?

REFLECT

- How would your life change if you could experience and appreciate the magic and the gifts in those moments?

- How many of those moments have been long forgotten in the recesses of your memory?
- What if you and your loved ones were able to share these memories – these magical moments – regularly remembering to celebrate this profound gift we call life?

This chapter will help you to open the treasure box of these memories. This book will teach you to discover those moments, savor them, and experience a whole new perspective on living your life. Frankly, all you need is a moment to remember and capture the magic in your life – including new magical moments as they are happening.

We make sense of our world through the stories we share with one another. We all know that children love to hear stories. Throughout history, life lessons and experiences have been shared through stories. These magical moments are mechanisms to teach, learn, motivate, and inspire those around you to evaluate and identify magical moments in their own lives. Happiness is contagious. Everyone wants to catch it. So to truly understand and appreciate the importance of magical moments, let's take the time to absorb the relationship between magical moments and our own lives.

What Is a Magical Moment?

A magical moment is a unique moment in our life. It can be a moment we experience right now, or it can be a memory from our past. Some are joyful, some sad, some inspiring, and some enormously challenging. Whatever the case may be, together these magical moments make up our life – our legacy in this world.

Remembering these moments can lift us out of our day-to-day routine to experience a deeper and more profound level of life – the sort of life of which we could only dream. These experiences are rich with emotion, deeper meaning, and extensive fulfillment. It's like opening a treasure box of history and finding the golden nuggets. We all have them.

Some are buried deeper than others. Some even have immense value that may go unrecognized at first, only to be discovered later. They are all there, just waiting to be uncovered. Consider the following magical moment that occurred at our family's dinner table. It illustrates the spontaneity of magical moments, but it also demonstrates how powerful these special opportunities can be.

Magical Moments – *A Family Tradition*

A guest sits with a questioning look: what is a magical moment? I turn to our twelve-year-old son Cristian and ask him, "Can you please tell our guest about magical moments?" He explains, "A magical moment is a special moment in your life – anytime in your life. When you have dinner with our family, you remember that moment and share it with everyone here."

"Who will start?" I asked.

My daughter speaks up. "I was afraid. We were driving in a scary part of Los Angeles. My mom said we should go. It was drizzling outside. I felt a chill up my back not only from the cold, but also from what I saw. So many of them under cardboard boxes; others were soaking wet just standing there with blank looks. I was grateful to pull into the secure parking lot for the Midnight Mission homeless shelter. We were in the heart of Skid Row. I was still nervous when we started serving dinner to them, so many homeless people. They kept coming through the line. I was tense. Then a young girl came through my line. She was cold and pregnant. Where was her coat? Did she have one? 'Do you have any dessert? I was hoping for just one cupcake.' I was stunned. She was as old as me. We didn't have cupcakes. In fact, there was no dessert at all. How could a teenage girl be here? I realized in a moment what my life would be like if I were homeless. I will never take my life for granted again."

It was my turn to speak. "Last week I found a thirty-year-old newspaper article about my father. He was a ballroom dancer, and the article was about his passion for dancing. After many years of severe illness, he recovered when he was sixty-five. He lived the final decade of his life determined to enjoy every moment. He had such a zest for life and having fun. He was a bit eccentric, and sometimes his hair dye would be too dark or his Old Spice men's cologne would be too strong. Yet he was the life, and fun, of anywhere he went. People loved his magnetic, loving, and care-free nature. That article reminded me to take time to do things just for the sheer fun, for the laughter, for the moment. His life was such a blessing in my life and this world."

My eighteen-year old son begins, "I had just finished my fifth bas-ketball game at the gym, and I was exhausted. I was walking out the door to go home when I heard someone call, 'Hey, Oliver – one more!' I had no idea that turning around could have led to my season being jeopardized. I played, and during that game I went for a layup. As I was falling back to the floor I felt my foot land on another shoe and rapidly twist and crack. I was helped to the nearby seats and lay down for about an hour. All I could think about was that split-second decision to play in that game. I could never undo that. One small decision could have just ended my whole basketball season. I went through a long, difficult rehabili-tation and luckily healed much faster than the doctor expected. I learned an important lesson that day that will serve me my whole life. I really have to stop and think about all decisions in my life before I make them. There are consequences to every action. Who knew that stepping back on that court could have changed my life forever?"

The rest of us shared our magical moments while my son's teen-age friend Austin was quiet, as he was most days with his basket-ball team. After everyone shared, it was his turn: "My magical moment was last week when I drove to the airport and picked up my father. He just finished his tour of duty in Afghanistan, and he is alive. I was so happy and grateful that he came home. He had many friends that didn't make it. Picking him up from the airport was the happiest day of my life."

We all paused. I said a silent prayer of gratitude, appreciating all the magic right there at my dinner table.

While we are sitting in traffic, or cooking dinner, or reflecting on our day, one young man is driving to the airport, thanking God that his father survived the war. He is being reunited with the most important person in his life, excited for the opportunity to once again embrace and look into the eyes of his loving father. Magical moments occur throughout the world every second of every day. We are all unique individuals with our own histories, experiences, and values. We each have our own story. Each of our magical moments reflects our individuality and creativity while providing the rich and colorful tapestries that cover our lives.

There are as many types of magical moments as there are people in this world. Your magical moments can be anything – a simple quiet moment alone watching a beautiful sunset, a celebration of a life moment with others, a personal moment of inspiration, overcoming grief, experiencing gratitude, a genuine belly laugh, or almost anything that moves you to a state of emotion, reflection, and warmth. It's a feeling of grace and connectedness to your life that transcends your day-to-day routine. It is your own sacred experience. You can feel it within, and when you do, it reverberates with every chord in your body.

There are bits of magic in our lives just waiting to be captured. These magical moments are all around us. These fleeting experiences are there to be appreciated. They are there for just an instant and can pass us by in the blink of an eye.

Oftentimes we appreciate the lessons in an experience long after they actually occur. Sometimes it takes time to understand the gifts in those moments. The time to reflect often shines a lens onto the meaning of the moment. We need to have faith that there are lessons and magic in every opportunity, even if we can't see, feel, or understand them at the time. We have to trust that the lessons will come with time and serve us when we need them the most.

During the day, our thoughts are generally occupied with asking and answering questions. We have experiences, we decide what they mean, and we then take action based on those meanings. We create many of our beliefs based on the meanings we give our life experiences. Just because we believe something doesn't necessarily mean that it is true.

Think back on the last time you told someone else, or yourself, a story about your life. What meaning did you give the story? How has that meaning affected your life? Is it a positive meaning or a negative meaning? Both? Then think days, weeks, or even months down the road. Did you ever reflect on the initial meaning you gave the moment, only to consider an entirely different significance later? This occurs because time offers the opportunity to reflect, translate, and evaluate the meaning behind the moments.

REFLECT

- How much magic is at your dinner table waiting to emerge?
- Think of a way that you and your loved ones can discover your most treasured memories together?
- Look back on a challenging moment in your life. Can you now find the lesson, gift and inspiration in it?

The Gift Magical Moments Give You

You may think to yourself, "Why should I really care about experiencing magical moments?" Magical moments not only enhance your life and offer you the opportunity to find happiness and enlightenment, but each moment is also a chance to learn about yourself and others. These opportunities offer you the occasion to notice what really makes you happy, pull you toward your purpose in life, and allow you to experience an intense feeling of love for yourself, for others, and for life. Magical moments push you to feel all the colors of the rainbow. But first we need to pause and reflect: What do I see in this moment? What do I hear? What am I feeling right now? From those experiences we can learn about our authentic self and what makes us unique in this world. We can begin to better understand our passions and even our challenges and search and find the magic in those moments that really inspire us.

As we fall into our daily routines, our senses get numbed by the day-to-day rat race. As our senses weaken, our lives can become dull and gray and we are less and less able to connect with the light that fuels us. If you are like me, you wake up each day with a long list of things you need to get done. As the day progresses, you start to feel satisfied as you check things off your to-do list. Yet, at the end of the day, an entirely new list appears and the cycle begins again. Sometimes we are more like "human doings," and we are challenged to find the time to really be a "human being." In those moments where we can just be, we open up a space to experience emotions and feel them again, even if it has been a long time since we allowed ourselves to just be and feel.

The gifts of magical moments are endless. They create peace and a sense of calmness in an otherwise tumultuous and stressful world. Your mind, body, and soul are pulled in different directions each and every day, affected and inflicted by the environment, humanity, and numerous other demands. But finding our magical moments offer a breath of fresh air, a release from the consistent stress we see, hear, and feel on a daily basis. Imagine a world filled with endless happiness, laughter, warmth, and meaning. One where you look to your left, to your right, up and down, and see nothing but comforting, sincere, and real surroundings which draw you in and uplift your heart and soul. These are just a few of the gifts a world with magical moments offers.

The Greater Good

Reconnecting to a life filled with magical moments is not only unbelievably fulfilling, it is also advantageous to both your life and the overall spirit and prosperity of humanity. Focus on magical moments and your life will not only feel different, it will be different, and that will resonate to others. But to reconnect to a fulfilling life, you must also align your actions and behaviors to those that support the greater good. As we awaken each morning and navigate the world, we are given the exciting opportunity to make a difference in the lives of those we touch. This could be the barista that serves you coffee, those people driving the cars around you, your employees or coworkers, and obviously your loved ones.

Every day you are offered the responsibility to enhance the world in which you live. Winston Churchill said, "We make a living by what we get, we make a life by what we give." Magical moments are gifts that can be given and shared with others. Buy the young lady in line behind you a cup of coffee, allow a few cars to go in front of you in heavy traffic, hold open the door for a stranger, or make time to read to your children or cook a nice meal for your husband or wife. These small but focused actions brighten the world and inspire others to do the same.

REFLECT

- When was the last time you did something for the greater good of this world without expecting anything in return?
- When was the last time you saw someone in need and actually did something about it?
- When was the last time you felt grateful for the opportunity to serve someone else?

- When was the last time you took steps to impact the greater good of humanity?

Some traditions teach that when you see someone in need, it is no coincidence. In that situation, you are in the best position to make the biggest difference. The belief is that such a person was put in your path because you have a responsibility to help them. How would your life change if you believed this principle? What if you were the person in need? Enhancing the greater good is opportunity driven. When you see the occasion to help another, it is your responsibility to grasp the chance and pay it forward. These are some of the most meaningful magical moments as they involve uplifting and improving the life of an individual who desperately needs it.

We are all opportunity creators. We are all pivotal pieces of the greater good. In fact, the greater good relies upon, even calls upon, each of us to play our part. The greater good is like a race without a finish line. It is a work in progress and constantly calls for each of us to do our best 100 percent of the time. There is always an individual or community in need, a hungry mouth to feed, legs that need support, a mind that is starving for direction, and a heart that requires warmth.

We Live in a Bubble – *Shelter on Skid Row*

> *I was very fortunate recently to bring my children to a homeless shelter in Los Angeles to serve meals to the homeless population. While there, the volunteer coordinator shared with us that about 30 percent of the homeless population on Skid Row have college degrees. After learning this information, my children and I had an amazing discussion about all the many unforeseen reasons people become homeless and how fortunate we are in our lives. In that magical moment together, we felt even more grateful for the opportunity to serve that day, and for the gift of our own lives.*

Magical moments allow us not only to offer gratitude but also to receive it. In moments like the one above, we are offered a valuable opportunity to distance ourselves from the comfort of our own lives and learn more about the lives of others. We helped serve food, but we were the ones who received the greatest gifts. We were offered insight, viewpoint, and in-depth knowledge of how we could help to prevent homelessness and uplift the people in that position. This impromptu and unexpected experience led to an increase in our family's desire to focus on finding a solution, while simultaneously addressing the problem.

The greater good is grounded in the notion that if we come together in a focused and dedicated manner, we can make an enormous difference in the lives of others. Whether we accept it or not, we are all in this together. As the lucky inhabitants of earth, we share the same resources and opportunities. No one person deserves any more of these than another. So when the exciting and meaningful opportunity arises to make change or alter the life of a person traversing difficult terrain, it is for the greater good to do so. Magical moments are the foundation for change. The greater good is not so great right now. Too many people squander the chance to take a moment to change a life or change the world we live in. But if you take the time personally to reconnect to a fulfilling life, you can begin to not only transform your life but also the lives of others.

$\mathcal{3}$

CHAPTER THREE

Shifting to a Life Filled with Magical Moments

I always think of each night as a song.
Or each moment as a song.
But now I'm seeing we don't live in a single song.
We move from song to song, from lyric to lyric, from chord to
chord. There is no ending here. It's an infinite playlist.

– David Levithan, Nick & Norah's Infinite Playlist

The Power in Your Mind, Body, and Spirit

Anthony Robbins has said, "Where focus goes energy flows." The shift to living a life of special and unique moments is found within your mind, body, and spirit. Change the way you think and feel, and what you welcome in your life, and you will exchange unfulfilling moments for exquisite ones. It starts with focusing on what needs to change and then diverting the energy flowing through your body in a dedicated and streamlined manner. The mind and body at work can fulfill and accomplish amazing results.

There is magic in your mind, your body, and your spirit right now. Opening this book, reading these words, being here right now. There is magic. You might ask: Where exactly is the magic? How do I find it? And then how do I use it to reinvent my purpose and my goal?

Tapping into your mind will begin the path to mastering your own life. Our minds process information and then create "maps" or belief systems that shape the way we view the world. For relevance in this book, this is when we create positive or negative meanings for the experiences in our lives. If we create a different meaning for an experience – a magical meaning – then we will experience life completely differently.

REFLECT

- When you have a challenging experience, start by asking yourself, "What does this mean?"
- Then proceed to ask, "What else can this mean?"
- You could even go further and ask, "What would have to happen for me to find the gift, lesson, and magical meaning in this experience?"

So to begin to shift, you first have to empower yourself and recognize that you are capable of making the necessary changes and give any situation the meaning you choose. If you desire to transform your life, then you are proficient and skilled to do so. The power is inherent in your mind, body, and spirit but calls for your dedication to tap into these powerful resources and then implement them into your traditions, rituals, and everyday practices.

Training Your Mind

So here we go. It is time to put the plan in motion and begin the shift. Your mind is a miracle. Most people believe that life happens outside their body. The truth is you experience life based on what you process in your mind. Everything that happens in your life is received through your sight, hearing, touch, taste, and smell. Your body then receives information through your senses and your mind processes it into your memories and meanings. Is it good or bad? Happy or sad? Funny or serious? Your mind decides what is important to remember and filters out the rest. Those memories define your life.

Two people can be at the same place at the same time and yet have completely different experiences and memories based on what information they let into their minds and the meaning they give that information. One may walk away with a sense of dissatisfaction and the other leave feeling as if he or she experienced a magical moment. Have you ever gone to a movie with a friend and left saying "that was awesome" and your friend said, "I hated it"? That's because the movie had different meanings for each of you. Your mind has tremendous power over determining the course of your life. Is this moment magical or horrible? Are you able to find the magic and the gifts in an experience, or do you generally default to what is wrong?

In those moments, your mind determines your beliefs. Tony Robbins teaches, "Beliefs have the power to create and the power to destroy. Human beings have the awesome ability to take any experience of their lives and create a meaning that disempowers them or one that can literally save their lives."

Have you ever met a person who said, "Bad things always happen to me"? Their mind will filter out most references to good things happening to them because that is not consistent with their belief. They will focus primarily on bad things happening to them to "prove" their belief, which will most likely lead to a victim mentality and a negative life.

Alternatively, have you ever met someone who said, "My life is beautiful and such a gift"? That person will tend to focus on gratitude and what is great about life, deleting most experiences that are not beautiful, which will lead toward a more positive and happy life. Positive people are attracted to positive attitudes and behaviors. If you generate a life filled with optimism and encouraging practices, like magnets people will be attracted to you and come into your life. Simply projecting your goals and desired outcomes into the world can prove to be a powerful manner of manifesting change and reaching goals.

Finding the Magic of It – *Woody's Story*

Choose Being Happy Over Being Right…
and You Will Be Right Every Time

Without getting too far out of the wheelhouse of magical moments, let me first say that I have found that magical moments can be simple and spontaneous as well as planned and created. Either way, for me, the magic is the lesson you get from that experience. So, what if you read this story, received the same lesson I did, and your life and the lives of others were enriched?

I learned that there is magic in almost everything, even in things that we feel hold us back or prevent us from being happy and fulfilled in our lives. Maybe it's the way someone acted years ago, and you have made it mean something that keeps you from having a relationship with him or her. It can be anything that you want it to be.

Okay, my magic moment came one day about twenty years ago when I least expected it. I was driving in the car with my father's third wife and was deep into my story of how my father's past treatment of his children had caused us much unhappiness. I was very self-righteous in my conversation. My story was that my father had four small children when he left and ran off with another woman. He never called except on the two most important days of the year – Christmas and our birthdays. These calls were awkward moments (back then, certainly not magic). I resented and blamed this man who was my father because I felt I only mattered to him on those two days, and he was supposed to be the most important person in my life.

So back to my stepmother and me having a magic moment...

She listened patiently and then paused and asked me, "Do you want to be right, or do you want to be happy?"

Immediately I responded, "When I am right, I am happy."

She said, "So how do you know if you are right?" Wow—that brought me another perspective. I had to think about it for a moment. Of course I know when I am right. When I feel "right," I am certain that life is supposed to be this way, regardless of the circumstances involved; however, feeling self-righteous wasn't making me feel good, even though I convinced myself it did. Simply put, my stepmother was giving me a lesson in how I could be happy.

The question she asked – "Do you want to be right, or do you want to be happy?" – changed my focus, and the possibility of magic taking place began. That question changed the meaning I associated with being "right" about things and led me to be more flexible as a way to be happier. Before that, it was about having a life in accordance with my rules about "what was right" and the way things were supposed to be.

I shifted my focus from "being right" to "being happy." This required that I find new meanings in situations by asking better questions. Then the magic of being happy could begin. I started to find or look for the gift or lesson in a situation. Sometimes we think that some situations are happening to us instead of for us. Frankly, I learned that life isn't always about getting what I want just because I feel that's the way it is supposed to be.

So for me this magic moment was in a car going down South Dixie Highway with my father's third wife. That ride in the car began many conversations with myself about creating a happy life. I realized that the only meaning anything has is the meaning you give it. It is my choice to find the gift.

In that car she asked me, "Can you think for a moment about how your father must feel every time he thinks about his choice to leave his four children? Do you ever think about how much his choice hurts him – so much so that he would do anything to avoid thinking about it? He only did what he had to do on the two days of the year, your birthday and Christmas, because every time he had to focus on you children it reminded him of what he had done. He was not proud of it."

I replied, "It's interesting to know that he shared that with you because he never shared that with any of his children. We all felt we did not matter."

She said, "I do know that your father is proud of you and what you have accomplished." When she said that, I actually remembered times he had told me he was proud of me. I had blown it off because I was making him wrong for the choice he had made years ago. I was beginning to see things differently...

I had an awakening... a breakthrough... a new possibility... a magic moment.

Maybe I had been right in blaming my dad for leaving, but I couldn't blame him for all the things that went wrong with my life. Maybe the opportunity was to see all I had gotten from his choice instead of focusing on what I was blaming him for. In that moment, we talked about how being ignored by my dad was maybe one of the reasons I tried so hard to matter and as a result had success in business. Maybe I needed to credit him for a part of that!

I am so thankful for that magic moment I shared with my stepmom. It's one I remind her of whenever we are together. My dad died almost ten years ago, and I still look at him differently because of this moment... it was truly magic. It changed my focus and beliefs about a story I had been telling myself for over thirty years.

A magic moment could have already happened to you as you read this. Look back and reflect on some of the areas in your life that have brought you pain, or try to remember choices people made that affected you emotionally. Ask yourself,

- *Do I want to be right, or do I want to be happy?*
- *What is the gift in this moment?*
- *What is amazing in my life right now because of this moment?*
- *Right now, what am I proud of in my life as a result of this moment?*
- *Who do I cherish in my life now because of this moment?*
- *How have I grown because of this moment?*
- *Where is the magic in this moment?*

You can have a magic moment right now from something in the past. You can choose to ask better questions and change the mean-

ing of events so that they empower you and free you from the need to be right. Instead, be happy.

For me, that question was a magic moment. It freed me. A new loving and empowering relationship with my dad began. I found out what could be great about a bad situation. In it I started a whole journey of discovery and found that the best in life is not what you get but who you become. Also, who you become is not as important as being happy in the process of becoming.

It is not what you get to keep but what you get to give that will bring you the fulfillment you desire. The secret of magic is looking for it in everything.

As I said earlier in the first chapter, we lead busy lives. Rarely do we have time to ask these important questions. This book is about pausing to find the magic in every moment, even our most challenging moments, and answering these important questions. Those are the moments that define us. When life is going well, it is easy to say, "I love my life. I am happy. I do the right thing. I live with integrity and strength." But life will test you. It is in those difficult experiences that we are challenged to test our beliefs. That is when it is critical to find the magic. It's there; you just need to have the right focus and ask the right questions. Training your mind to focus on your magical moments is a skill. It takes a bit of conditioning and focus. But once you do, it becomes a habit and second nature.

REFLECT

- What are some of your most important beliefs?
- What meanings have you given to some of the most important experiences in your life?
- Who have you become as a result of those experiences?
- How would your life be if you changed those meanings to something more positive and inspiring?

- What do you think about most during the day?
- Knowing that "where focus goes energy flows," what do you focus on most in life?

Who Are You?

As you train your mind, you will find yourself searching for important answers and reflecting on your life's direction. First and foremost, consider evaluating exactly who you are. This may seem obvious, but if you are unaware of who you are, you will be at a disadvantage when you attempt to change. If you ask someone who they are, they will usually describe their position or their possessions.

- "I am a mother."
- "I am a teacher."
- "I am a salesperson."
- "I am a surfer."
- "I am a homeowner."

While true, these definitions can limit our ability to live a full and meaningful life. The true magic in each of us is not in what we do or what we own, but in who we really are at our core. Our fabric is what makes us special. Many of us seek to live a fulfilling life, yet rarely do we stop to think about what that really means or who we need to be to feel fulfilled.

Spending time alone is a perfect way to explore who we are and to realize the magical moments we can create in our lives and in the lives of others. Would your magical moments have a different meaning if you had a different identity? Of course they would. A story of an accident victim would have a different moral if it was written by someone who constantly focuses on what they cannot do in life due to their injuries instead of a person who inspires other challenged individuals to reach for all they want in the world. One would be a story of despair and the other would be a story of courage and inspiration. What do your stories say about who you are?

As you begin your transformation to a life filled with magical moments, you first have to understand who you are, not what you have. Consider the notion that the definition of who you are is not controlled by what you own, where you live, what you drive, or what you do for a living. The truth is that you are the totality of your heart, mind, and soul. Those unbelievably beautiful and non-tangible pieces of your fabric cannot be purchased, sold, or acquired. The strength and spirit of your heart, mind, and soul are what make or break you. They are the pieces that allow you to reach goals, succeed in life, and make an undeniable difference in the lives of others. The greater good relies upon your decision to define who you are not by what you have but by what you have inside. To build magical moments and shift to a life filled with happiness and immeasurable success, you have to first completely reinvent your definition of who you are.

REFLECT

- Who are you?
- Who are you really?
- Who would you need to be to live a meaningful life, be happy, and reach your dreams?
- What would have to happen now for you to be that person?

Awakening Your Spirit

Noticing, experiencing, and appreciating the magical moments in your life every day is a skill. In mastering any skill, you first need to learn techniques and then apply and practice them every day to condition them into your mind and body. It takes conditioning and commitment. After some time, you realize that it is no longer what you "do" anymore; it is who you "are."

Whether we realize it or not, our expression of our own magical moments reaches a deep part of our spirit. They rekindle our memories. People who hear our stories are inspired and moved to remember their own. When we share our joy, others search for their own joy. When we share our sorrow, we touch others' hearts and they remember their own times of sadness. When we share our pain, others are moved to find their compassion and remember their own healing experiences. These stories connect all of us and remind us that we are united in many ways. Far beyond the air we breathe or the space we occupy, we truly are united in spirit.

Try this…

Pause now and take a moment to remember a time in your life that was special and memorable for you. It could be any moment, with family, friends, alone, in nature, with God – any wonderful memory.

Breathe that in…

What did you see?

See where you were at that time. See the people around you. See everything in your world at that moment. Let that vision become brighter and envelop you in the moment. Be in that moment now.

What did you hear?

Hear the sounds in that moment. Hear the sounds of everything around you. Hear the voices of the people with you. Hear your own thoughts from that moment. Let those sounds become louder now.

What did you feel?

Feel the feelings you felt at that moment. Feel them radiate and deep within you. Let them radiate through your body right now.

What was the magic in that moment for you?

Pause and fully enjoy the experience. Truly appreciate that unique moment in your life.

What did that moment mean for you?

How has that moment served you in your life?

Appreciate the magic in that moment and the many magical moments you have had in your past, have right now, and will have in your future. This simple act of awakening your spirit and reflecting on your inherent feelings when magic moments do appear allows you the exciting occasion to connect with them more often. Your spirit is a driving force in locating and manifesting these magical moments. It is like gas for the car. You are the vessel; your spirit is what makes you run. Once you invigorate your inner excitement – your spirit – you will once again locate your enthusiasm for life and find that magical moments are everywhere, ready for you to tap into them and introduce them as an integral part of your own daily life.

REFLECT

- When do you take time to pause and think about the memorable moments in your life?
- When was the last time you shared those moments with the people in your life?
- Are you able to find the gifts and lessons in each experience, or do you tend to focus on the negative?
- What would have to happen so you can regularly tap into and awaken the joyful and grateful spirit and experiences within you?

Conditioning Your Body

Once the mind is awake, the body will follow. Your body is a miracle. Right now approximately one hundred trillion cells in your body are acting together to keep you alive. Each cell does a few million things per second to keep functioning, and they all started from one cell. Scientists still can't figure out how one cell divides up into so many different parts of our body. More miraculous is that all of those cells work together in synchronicity, coordinating their every activity to give you life every day.

We have all heard the saying "monkey see, monkey do." This is particularly useful to illustrate that before we act, we think. A thought is introduced into our head, and then our mind fires off directions to the body to act, react, or simply move. Thus, for every thought we have, there is an automatic corresponding reaction in your body. That is why our analysis began with a discussion of the power of the mind and the steps to awaken the spirit. The body is what does the heavy lifting from a literal sense. But the interconnectivity between mind and body is endless. Just like your mind, your body has its own memory. Our bodies can remember specific areas of pleasure and pain, sometimes long after our intellectual memory of such events fades. Consider the following magical moment demonstrating the unbelievable connection between body and mind.

Squeeze Your Fist, Feel the Energy – *A Triathlete's Story*

The big black Sharpie graced my arm and my back leg with the number 241. My bike was in place with my helmet resting loosely on top, my running shoes carefully set near the aisle. I squeezed one leg, then another, and then my arms into the skintight wetsuit and placed the colored cap on my head. All set! As I walked to the Pacific Ocean's edge I began my longstanding tradition of squeezing my fist before and after each race—my physical ritual to remember each and every past race in the palm of my hand. My body responded accordingly and flooded my mind and spirit with all of my past triathlons—race after race after race. Seeing myself cross the finish line, hearing the cheers of the crowd, feeling that exhilaration of another successful race completed, I filled my mind with intensely focused magical moments of challenge and success as I had done many times before. The horn blew signaling the start, and I relaxed my fist and dove into the ocean. The flood of memories engaged my mind, fueled my spirit, energized my body, and sent me sailing across the water with the finish line in my mind long before it was in actual sight.

This athlete floods her memory with her successes from past races. She recreates the intensity of those moments by remembering what she saw, what she heard, and what she felt in those race moments. While intensifying those moments in her mind, she squeezes her fist to create a physical anchor in her body. This anchor creates a memory of those magical moments in her body. So anytime she squeezes her fist, her body's memory will go back to feeling the intensity of those race moments, even if she doesn't remember the specifics. Her body will remember for her.

I know many athletes who use this emotional flood and anchoring technique to get in a peak state prior to starting an athletic event. Great speakers and leaders use similar techniques to get into a peak-energized state before leading their audiences. They take time to fill their minds, bodies, and spirits with magical moments to inspire them. I recently even used this flooding and anchoring technique with my nine-year-old son to teach him how to get in a positive peak state before he gave his "Scholar Speak" speech to his third-grade class!

Mind and body are seamlessly connected. They are part of the same infrastructure, working in a synchronistic manner to effectuate the same goals. As we redefine our goals to help produce magical moments in this world, our mind and body will begin to fall into place. As our thoughts become actions, and our positive actions become meaningful habits, magical moments will manifest themselves in abundance. Conditioning does not occur overnight, but small changes often lead to large ones. The highly successful and inspiring entrepreneur and teacher, Keith Cunningham, reminds us, "Ordinary things done consistently create extraordinary results." It's the little things we do each day that can shift our lives in an entirely new direction. Thus, we strive to start now in hopes of reaching our goals tomorrow. So with that in mind, let's shift our focus, along with our goals, to recognizing those types of moments for which we should strive.

Shifting our Focus to Our Moments

Magical moments come in different shapes and sizes. As we continue our journey, we will categorize our moments into general areas of life that will motivate you to evaluate and reflect on those areas in your own life to create more magical moments. But before we can do that, let's discuss the emotions and traits that will help you to lay the groundwork for these moments. These are the feelings, sentiments, and passions that run through your body, maintaining your heart and soul as you experience life. As you increase the levels of these sensations, you will find a life better positioned to welcoming an amazing amount of magical moments.

The Magic of Emotions

Underneath every magical moment lies an unbelievable and passionate amount of emotion. Helen Keller said, "The best and most beautiful things in the world cannot be seen or even touched. They must be felt with the heart." Your whole life is experienced in your mind through what is received and then perceived through your senses and felt through your heart and soul. Think about it—your whole life is processed in your mind through what you see, hear, feel, smell, and taste. When was the last time you really appreciated the magic of your mind? Your mind is the compass for you to navigate and truly feel your emotions. These same emotions allow you to experience joy, relieve stress, feel unbridled happiness, and cope with sorrow when it occurs. Emotion is the splash of color in an otherwise black-and-white world. There is enormous magic in emotion, and many of the magical moments we experience in life are manifested in our emotional responses.

When you experience a magical moment in the present, your whole being is taken to a lighter more blissful place. Even when you experience a memory of a past magical moment, you also can experience that lighter, more peaceful and more joyful place. Virginia Woolf said, "I can only note that the past is beautiful because one never realizes an emotion at the time. It expands later, and thus we don't have complete emotions about the present, only about the past."

As you will learn in the following chapters, living and remembering more and more of your magical moments will bring you even more peace, joy, and success while also relieving stress, anxiety, and frustration. Magical moments will lift you out of your day-to-day state of being into a higher state of consciousness to truly live an exceptional, extraordinary, and blissful life.

Emotions change your state of consciousness, conditioning a new paradigm and allowing more meanings to flow from experiences, thus producing more meaningful and magical moments. What if you could change the way you feel anytime you wanted? In choosing your emotions and allowing them to pave the way to more purpose and meaning in life, you have the unparalleled opportunity to accomplish just that. It is there right in front of you. It is time to celebrate our emotions and pause to experience the miracle of life.

REFLECT

- What three positive emotions do you feel most each week?
- How is your life impacted when you feel these?
- What three negative emotions do you feel most each week?
- How is your life impacted when you feel these?

Gratitude – When was the last time you truly felt grateful? Can you remember a time in your life when someone made a significant impact – a game changer – and they never really knew it, and may not know it even now? Gratitude is the act of expressing appreciation. It could be a few kind words, a thank-you card, or a hug or kiss. You should remain grateful for everyone who has touched your life. Even for the challenging people, as they helped to form both you and your story. It could be a teacher, employer, family member, or friend. Maybe even a stranger, a sales associate, or your mailman. There always lies the exciting opportunity to show gratitude and thank others for their actions.

In an episode of Oprah's Lifeclass, life strategist Tony Robbins says that gratitude packs a powerful punch against anger and fear. "Fear is why we don't take action, and anger is why we get stuck," Tony says. "You can't be grateful and angry simultaneously. You can't be fearful and grateful simultaneously. So it's really the reset button."

The great thing about being grateful is that it leads you to take the valuable steps of scanning your life for people, places, things, and moments that are magical. Think about what evokes gratitude in you. Why are you grateful? What specifically about each of those things is a lesson, a gift, and a magical moment? Even our darkest moments give us the gift of knowing the difference between dark and light, bad and good, sad and happy.

In that same Lifeclass program, Oprah says that each leader's definition of gratitude reminds us that gratitude is the ultimate spiritual solution to help us connect to something greater.

REFLECT

- What would have to happen for you to fully appreciate all the gifts in your life?
- What would have to happen for you to realize that you have gifts in your life?

We all have been given gifts – some big, others small. Regardless, it is our duty to identify the gift-givers and show appreciation for their actions. As you take the time to show greater gratitude toward others, you will unlock the doors and open the windows for magical moments to creep in. Appreciation attracts special moments and allows those moments to play pivotal roles in manifesting happiness in your life.

Love – Love paves the way for unbelievable moments. When was the last time you truly felt love? It doesn't have to be romantic but rather the sensation of love within your whole body, mind, and spirit. It doesn't happen every day, but when it does, it is a truly remarkable feeling. Love illuminates the world, brightening it and infusing it with a guiding light. For those who are lucky to feel this emotion every day, life is better for it. To love and be loved is not always easy and often calls for you to take down the walls and other obstacles you've potentially created to stop it from shining through. Once you are available for love, you will find it in so many different ways.

Magical moments thirst for love. Love is satisfying, purifying, and quenching. Love offers relief and allows magical moments to grow exponentially. As you love more, your life will become infused with those special moments that only love can manifest. Think about the happiest moments in your life. Were they shared with a loved one? A friend or family member? Magical moments are usually lined with a radiant feeling of love. Love supports the world and allows your life to be one that changes it as well.

REFLECT

- When was the last time you felt love?
- What would have to happen to take a moment to give love to someone else or yourself right now?

Joy – Pure, unadulterated happiness. Joy is a flood of happiness tied directly to a single moment. As we experience joy, we are better positioned to welcome more magical moments. With joy, the trick is identifying exactly what facets of your life allow the floodgates of happiness to open.

Oftentimes we forget just how important joy is to our lives. Sure, we know happiness is vital. But what about excessive happiness? The kind that is uncontrollable, generally unexpected, and without boundaries? Finding joy and celebrating it consistently ensures it comes back and often will position your life to welcome even more magical moments. It is usually the intersection of where happiness elevates to joy that a remarkable magical moment occurs. Work hard to locate happiness, but dedicate yourself tirelessly to raise happiness to joy.

REFLECT

- When was the last time you truly felt joy?
- When was the last time you said, "I really feel happy"?
- What would have to happen for you to feel joy right now?

Fun – We all want to have fun. Fun is the place where your activities are lined with happiness. Laughter is a great medicine and usually goes hand-in-hand with fun. When was the last time you belly-laughed? You know, the kind of laugh that is so intense you feel sore for hours after. If you have to think about the answer, it is not often enough. Locating fun is easy. Begin by creating a list of the activities or moments you consider to be fun. Then schedule those events into your daily life. At least a couple of times per week you should schedule fun.

Once you do that, you will find a distinct and direct correlation between having fun and creating magical moments. Fun is the place where your guard is down, the normal stressors of everyday life are diminished, and your heart is open for laughter to slide in. Far too often we trade fun for work, stress, and "productive" activities. But once you begin to schedule fun religiously, you will find that magical moments will prevail often.

REFLECT

- When was the last time you belly-laughed?
- What in your life is fun right now?
- What would have to happen for you to schedule fun in your life this week?

Passion – Think about what really gets you going. What does passion mean to you? When was the last time you felt passion? We can feel passion for something we do or someone we love. Often we feel passion when we are engaging in our true purpose in life. It's the experience of not only doing something but also feeling it deeply within our core. Passion is a strong and barely controllable emotion. It is a longing, something we have to have, and something we cannot live without.

REFLECT

- What are you passionate about?
- When was the last time you truly felt passion?
- What was the magic and gift in the moment?
- What would have to happen to feel that again in your life now?

Passion is reserved for those special people and activities that induce a feeling of intense love. When you fully partake in activities or surround yourself with people you are passionate about, you will find that magical moments abound. Similar to having fun, once you identify those people, places, and activities that transport you to a place of passion, find time on a weekly basis to build these exciting opportunities into your schedule. Passion is special; it is medicine for the soul. Have you taken your medicine today?

Peace – Many of our day-to-day lives are filled with stress. It affects our body, our conditioning, and our overall feeling of stability and comfort. As our life vibrates at enormously high levels, it becomes difficult to feel at peace. Life is experienced in our mind, body, and spirit. There is peace already within us; we just need to pause to experience it and allow it to overtake the feelings of anxiety and stress encompassing our lives.

REFLECT

- When was the last time you truly felt at peace in your life?
- What would have to happen for you to disconnect from your busy life and take a moment to breathe deeply and feel the peace already within you?

Peace is not a place easily obtained. It is a destination we can only reach if we turn off the distractions in our life. It calls for us to disconnect with the outside world and reconnect with our innermost thoughts. Once we can accomplish this and put the rest of our lives to sleep, we can begin to connect with those people and goals that generate happiness and a sense of calm. Magical moments require you to focus on the purist of thoughts and emotions. They connect with your life only when you disconnect from those interruptions and agitations that act as obstacles to peace. It takes focus, dedication, and a determined effort to invite peace into your life by reducing disturbances and interferences. So find time each day to be alone, and push the stop button on the commotions that disturb your peace. Once you do that, your mind, body, and soul will be better positioned to connect with magical moments.

Inspiration – When was the last time you truly felt inspired? Inspiration is the process of being mentally stimulated to do or feel something, especially in a creative manner. Inspiration is that deep-down urge you feel that tugs at your soul and opens you to respond by acting on it. It may not occur every day, even every week, but when you feel inspired, it is essential that you scratch the itch. In each of our lives, there are activities and people who inspire us. It could be a moment in nature, a song, an event, a family member or friend, even a mentor or coach. They push you to feel that inner drive and determination to reach higher and go farther than otherwise imaginable.

REFLECT

- What inspires you?
- When was the last time you truly felt inspired?
- What did you see, feel, hear, and experience in that moment?
- What would have to happen for you to feel inspired again?

We should all have the ability to pinpoint those people or activities that manifest inspiration. For me, my husband and my children inspire me to work hard and carry myself through life in a positive and morally strong manner. I look to them and hope they inject this attitude into their own lives. Inspiration is a deeply personal emotion that requires you to evaluate your life and then identify those small yet powerful pieces that move you to a place of extensive stimulation. Only then will you encourage and motivate more magical moments to appear.

Sorrow – As much as we don't want to think about it, life carries sadness, sorrow, and grief. If dedicated to finding happiness, the vast majority of your life will be happy. But there will be times, moments, and instances where you lose a loved one, run right into failure, or fall short of your goals. All emotions serve us, even the challenging ones. Sorrow is just one of the players in the game of life. But sorrow gives rise to magical moments as well. It doesn't mean it is a useless emotion just because it coincides with pain and hurt. Sorrow allows you the valuable opportunity to assess your life experiences and also provides contrast to the more positive emotions in your life. Sorrow forces you to gauge and calculate the role your current emotions play in the overall story of your life.

REFLECT

- When was the last time you experienced intense sorrow?
- What did that mean for your life?
- What else could it mean for your life?
- What were the gifts and lessons in that experience?

Think about what caused this feeling of sorrow, and consider how it serves you and how you will face sorrow the next time around. Life will present sorrow, but that doesn't mean you have to stay there or create more of it. Magical moments are created when you embrace your sorrow and use it to grow, cope, and heal. Consider the following magical moment and how it gives rise to hope and resilience.

Resilience – *A Moment of Gratitude for a Doctor's Gift of Time*

Family strife. Family conflict. Tension. Anger. Disintegration.

In the eyes of a child, there is no way out.
My eyes watching.
My ears hear.
My body feels nothing, but really feels everything.
Tired. Scared. Alone.
My voice silent.

In the eyes of a teen, finding a way out.
Escape.
Release.
Where is home?

I left home in my teens. My parents had gone through a painful divorce. I lived with my father and watched his alcoholism destroy his life until he was put into rehab. Who was I now? Where to turn? Friends? Family – what family? My mom closed the door and I was on my own.

Dr. Muller came into my life by chance. I knew I needed some help. As I look back thirty-five years, the memories have faded. Sitting in his office session after session, he looked so formal in his dress pants and collared shirts. I had no money, but he worked it out… small payments here and there. I think I finally paid him years later… I hope I did…

Resilient. He said, "You are one of the lucky few in life who are resilient." He believed in me. He gave me hope—one of the few people who did. I would sit in the sacred space of his office and feel safe. In that little office in Novato, California, my heart opened and the pain and strife of a hurting child and the sorrows of a lost teen poured out safely within those walls.

I remember thinking he was so formal and so "square." Yet he cared for me with his words, his stories, and his questions. His care and his time lifted a young girl from a painful childhood to a promising adulthood.

Hope.
Courage.
Strength.
Inspiration.

My eyes seek, look, and see.
My ears pause and listen intently.
My body is healthy.
Energized. Grateful. United.
My voice speaks and inspires.

Resilience. Yes, I am resilient, and now thirty-five years later I am so much more. Your gift of wisdom, time, and care pointed me in the right direction to have a life, a beautiful life. My magical moments in your office have created such magic in my life, the lives of my children, and the lives of so many others.

I am not even sure if he knows how much his lessons and gifts still serve my life. Dr. Francis Muller, this magical moment is for you as a moment of gratitude for all you have done for me, and I am sure for all you have done for countless others.

Resilience can be the product of responding to sorrow and other challenging emotions. You can internalize the pain and allow it to define your attitude, or you can deal with the sorrow and be stronger and wiser for it. Take the time to identify sorrow, accept it, and then utilize this powerful emotion as an opportunity to learn, heal, and create even more magical moments. Finding the gifts and magic in our most challenging times in life requires courage, strength, and faith.

Shifting to a life filled with magical moments is the result of understanding your emotions and recognizing the value they carry. Each emotion offers yet another opportunity to create a magical moment. You will find that there is a meaningful and direct correlation between showing gratitude, inviting love, experiencing fun, knowing joy, living with passion, focusing on peace, feeling inspired, and coping with sorrow and other challenging emotions in a healthy manner. By doing so, you will inspire others in your life to do the same and will plant the seeds for magical moments to grow within you and all around you. Shifting to a life filled with magical moments is a choice. It is a gift only you can give to yourself, and it is one that will ultimately pay you back in excess. These amazing magical moments are yours for the taking; Let's begin to capture them now.

4

Capturing Your Magical Moments

*What I like about photographs is that
they capture a moment that's gone forever,
impossible to reproduce*

– Karl Lagerfeld

With an understanding of those emotions and opportunities that produce an inspiring and optimistic environment for the creation of magical moments, let's shift our focus to capturing those amazing moments when they develop within your life. As fast as magical moments appear, with the blink of an eye they are gone. But the memories of them don't have to fade. You have the ability to capture and preserve these magical moments if you simply take the exciting opportunity to conserve and protect them for future enjoyment.

You Are Already a Storyteller

Every magical moment is a story. And you are already a capable and talented storyteller. Every time you tell someone about your life, you are telling a story and sharing a wonderful magical moment with him or her. We often have these conversations with ourselves. When was the last time you started a sentence similar to one of these?

> *"Yesterday I watched the most inspiring movie!"*
> *"Last night, my son and I had a heart-to-heart talk."*
> *"I finally resolved that challenge at work."*
> *"I have a friend with cancer."*
> *"My life has lost its spark."*
> *"I need some advice; here is what happened..."*
> *"Wow, I can't believe..."*
> *"I shouldn't or I should..."*

Any sentence about your life experience is the beginning of one of your stories. You are the medium, the surrogate, through which magical moments are passed from you to another. Every time you share a story about yourself or another, you open the door for a magical moment to be preserved or passed on. Magical moments are meant to be shared. They are communal, collective, and should never be kept under a cloak or behind a closed door.

Now it's time for you to find the magic, the special meaning, and the lessons the magical moments in your life can offer to others. Capturing your magical moments is easy. There are endless possibilities for finding the magic in your life. It is as easy as a mere thought, a brief pause in your day, or a few minutes of reflection. You may enjoy having a specific time each day that you devote to your magical moments. Some people love to reflect while in a certain special place. Others love sharing magical moments with other people. Music, sounds, pictures, sensations, tastes and special aromas can all be associated with your magical moments. Sometimes the best way to discover and appreciate your magical moments is in the silence of your mind. All of these techniques will serve to fill your mind, your spirit, and your body with the energy, joy, and gratitude your magical moments give your life. Just discover what works for you.

Remember, with the gift of memory and the ability to speak, you are well positioned to capture and then share moments that can inspire and influence the lives of others. It can be a disservice to others to keep special stories and magical moments hidden within your heart and soul. Magical moments can gain life and meaning when communicated to others. They are timeless and can literally change the world, one person at a time. You are the storyteller and the story-sharer that can take these moments and display them to the world, making a magnanimous difference to us all.

A Moment's Pause

At any point in your day, stopping to pause and remember a moment or two holds a space in your memory for that magic. It is a beautiful and simple way to fill your mind with magical moments. At any moment in time, you can pause and ask yourself, "What is a magical moment in my life? What's another one? And another?" Fill your mind with magical moments for a few seconds or a few minutes each day. While doing this, take yourself back to those moments. Fill your mind with what you felt, what you saw, and what you heard until your whole being is enveloped in those memories.

I have small signs posted around my house and on my desk to remind me of magical moments I hold dear to my heart. "What's another magic moment in your life?" "Life is not measured by the number of breaths we take but by the number of moments that take our breath away." "We don't remember days, we remember moments." They also are a constant cue to take the necessary time to capture magical moments. Creating and capturing magical moments is a concerted effort, a necessary regimen to which you can dedicate your life. Creating magical moments is like taking vitamins, working out, spending time with your family and loved ones, or even sleeping. Like these essential tasks, you have to schedule them into your daily routine.

Schedule the time to capture your magical moments. Try this: at the end of each day, find ten minutes of peace and time alone to reflect on your day. Survey where you were and whom you met. Consider those conversations and the meanings behind them. Think about the choices you made, the actions you took, and the consequences of those actions.

David Simon, MD, was the co-founder, CEO, and medical director of the Chopra Center for Wellbeing. Dr. Simon was dedicated to creating a healing healthcare system that encompasses the emotional, spiritual, as well as physical health of the individual. Dr. Simon taught, "Recapitulation, the technique of reviewing your choices and experiences at the end of each day, is a valuable technology for enhancing your communication skill set and keeping your heart free from toxicity." By putting on your investigative hat and studying your daily activities and interactions, you will find the ability to capture magical moments you hadn't even realized occurred.

Green Gables – *A Bride's Story*

My friend was sitting with me just as I was about to walk out onto the veranda at Green Gables. She said, "Here is my one piece of advice. Throughout this afternoon and evening stop to take mental snapshots. I know there is a photographer here, but these pauses are different. These are your special magical moments in time that you will engrain in your memory for a lifetime."

I walked out onto the veranda and the music started. In that moment, I paused and took my first mental snapshot. All eyes were on me. The most important people in my life were smiling, and I cherished their presence. I heard birds singing overhead. I paused to put my hands on my heart, and I really felt my heart beating. As I walked down the aisle, I could feel the warm sun on my shoulders.

It's remarkable. I only paused for about thirty seconds to take that mental snapshot, and yet now anytime I put my hands on my heart, my whole body remembers and feels the energy of love from that moment.

Mental snapshots promote the exciting proposition that magical moments not only occur when you aren't thinking about them, but – with a little reflection – they can be captured and passed on to others in a helpful and meaningful manner. So take the time to turn your mind into a high-resolution camera and examine your life so you can take those mental snapshots that will become important moments in your own life.

REFLECT

- How does your environment remind you to find joy every day?
- What mental snapshots do you have from your life?
- How have those moments shaped your life?
- What are the gifts and lessons from those moments?

One-Sentence Magical Moments

A magical moment can be captured in a story, and it can also be just as powerful when captured in one sentence. Sometimes the essence of a magical moment is best expressed in simple ways, in a sentence or two. They do not have to be longwinded or carry heavy explanations. Think of a quote. The beauty of a quote is its simplicity and punch. It is quick, easy, and leaves a lasting memory in the minds of its readers or hearers. So begin to consider your one-sentence magical moments.

We can have brief moments that have profound memories. Seeing a beautiful sunset, listening to the laughter of children, feeling the raindrops on our face. Each of those moments is simple yet powerful. Sometimes even the most significant parts of our life, our larger magical moments, can be best captured with just a sentence.

The Mustangs – *A Basketball Team's Magical Year*

During my son's last year of high school, he played varsity basketball. Being the team mom for his varsity basketball team gave me the special privilege of spending a lot of time with the players at various tournaments and games. I was blessed that they all knew me and at times welcomed me into their sacred circle. This team was special. Their bond was unlike any other I had seen on a sports team. These boys really loved each other and cared for each other like family—on and off the court. At the end of the year, we put together a video documentary of their season. I asked each of them for their magical moment. Like many teenagers, their words to adults, including me, were few. Yet those magical moments, many of which were only one sentence, captured the essence of their basketball experience as part of the Mustangs. Many adults, including me, who tend to use far too many words, can learn a lot from this group of teens about expressing and capturing what is important in life.

"My magical moment was in the locker room after the last game where we all shared how much we mean to each other."

"My magical moment was my whole year with this team, who really are my family."

"My magical moment was when my mom first put a basketball in my hand when I was a child."

"My magical moment was when coach first noticed me as a player in my freshman year and really made me feel special."

"My magical moment was when I realized that basketball is \a metaphor for life."

"My magical moments were more off the court when we all spent time together, especially now knowing we are all moving on to other parts of the country for college and may never all be together at once again."

Each of these simple yet impactful sentences reflects an extraordinary moment in each player's life. They quickly get to the crux of the experience and leave little to expand on. So, like the team members above, consider what events or experiences in your life could be summed up by just a couple of sentences. I'm willing to bet they end up being some of the most important and meaningful events you experienced.

REFLECT

- Can you remember a brief moment that you still hold in your heart?
- When was the last time you had a smile on your face?

- When was the last time you felt a tear on your cheek, the sun on your face, saw a rainbow, or heard someone say "I love you"?

Seven-Minute Magical Moment Stories

Often we focus our efforts on locating happy times. We forget that through sadness and challenge, some of life's most impactful lessons are forged. To this point, we have discussed the unbelievable power in telling a story. People leave feeling engaged, inspired, and highly motivated. But what about focusing on the story of your own life? Is there ever a time when you stop to identify those difficult moments in your life and simply reflect upon them?

A couple of years ago I attended a storytelling event where Bo Eason, a former NFL standout, Broadway playwright and performer, and outstanding performance/story coach, shared a great exercise that I use to capture my own magical moments. It is very simple. Your task is to write for seven minutes straight. Your goal is to focus on a memory and write anything – bad or good, grammatically correct or not, partial sentences, phrases…whatever shows up is perfect. Let your mind be free to recall the memory in any way that flows onto the paper. If you are done before seven minutes, great! If you go a little longer, great! Anything you write is perfect. Just keep writing for seven minutes.

Here's the initial catch. When we think of magical moments in our life, most of us go to the moments when we were most proud, when we felt great, and when we were celebrating. Instead, as you start these seven-minute stories, I want you to write about your most challenging moments – the moments that may have caused you pain, sadness, or grief. It is in these challenging moments that we can learn our greatest life lessons. As you write, allow whatever you remember or feel to pour onto the paper without editing or judging. This is your private story and no one needs to read it. It is a gift for you.

After you are done, take a moment to reflect on what you wrote. What does this story mean to you? What were the gifts and the magic in that moment?

Sometimes when we experience challenge, we can't always appreciate the lessons and gifts in that moment. Often our gratitude and the gifts from those moments don't show up until later in our lives. This exercise is one way to discover and capture the magic in those life moments. I now have several journals filled with these moments that serve as a memoir of my life.

Here is an example of one of my seven-minute magical moments:

Morning Tea – *A Mother's Stories*

It's 8:30 a.m. My kids have finally left for school and I am again so grateful that my seventeen-year-old drives my daughter to school. I pause to finish a cup of green tea, sit at my desk, and reach for the large book leaning up against my bed frame. I say to myself, "Wow – so many years, so many days, so many moments." As the book flips open, I can see the pages and pages that tell the multitude of stories that make up my life. I select purple from my pile of multicolored pens and open the book to the next blank page. I look at my clock, giving myself the gift of seven minutes. As the second hand reaches twelve, I start to write...

I am sixteen years old, my dad is ill, and I really need a job. The school knows the situation and will allow me to work for school credit to graduate. There is a posting at the local gas station. I tell this to a group of friends, and the boys in the group say, "You can't do that job. You are a girl and you wouldn't last a day."

I felt such fire in my words as I said, "Yes I can! YES I can!" I then marched down to the Shell gas station. It was the biggest gas station in the city with mostly full-serve islands. They hired me. I was determined to make it work. "Fill it up? Check your oil? How about your tires?" I had my regulars.

The mechanic Jerry scared me. Someone once told that he was an ex-con who had killed someone. He kept to himself most of the time. I knew he was watching me.

I look up; four minutes have passed, three to go.

It was a Friday morning in the summer. It was really hot outside and I was sweating as I finished serving a long line of cars. Jerry looked up at me. "Hey, Sissy, I bet you can't put that car on that lift and change that tire." I recall my reaction. First I felt disbelief. Whereas I was afraid of Jerry before, now I just felt that familiar fire. "Yes I can! YES I can." I walked over and picked up the car keys, got in, and drove the car over the lift. I got out of the car and checked its position. There was a big switch on the wall and I walked over to it. I didn't dare look at Jerry or the other mechanic. Up the car went on the huge airlift. I used the air gun to take off the lug nuts. It was so powerful that I gripped it really tight. I remember the beads of sweat on my forehead. I completed the task, lowered the car, and drove it to the holding area. Jerry nodded his head at me. "Good job, Sissy." I passed Jerry's unspoken test and earned his respect. I changed many tires. I completed many oil changes. At my auto maintenance class at school, I successfully took apart and put back together a transmission for my final.

"YES I can!" – my mantra for life. It has carried me through more challenges than I can write here. Suffice it to say, I graduated from the Boalt Hall School of Law at the University of California, Berkeley, without ever having an undergraduate degree. All because someone said, "No, you can't go to law school without going to college first." It is such a gift to realize in writing that

story, how one moment in a corridor at high school with a group of friends can impact your whole life...

I look at the clock again. Eight minutes have passed. I close my book, put it back in its sacred spot next to my bed frame, and begin my day.

REFLECT

- When could you schedule seven minutes to write about a challenging time in your life?
- What gifts and lessons could you possibly uncover by experiencing this seven-minute magical moment exercise?
- What would it mean to you and your family to have a memoir of moments in your life that were special, magical, and meaningful to you?
- What would it mean for you if you had such a memoir from those in your life who have passed on?

Press Record

There are so many easy ways to capture your magical moments. For example, my mobile phone came with a voice memo application, and smartphones and computers offer numerous recording applications that you can download. Install the best program on your smartphone or take the time to purchase a digital voice recorder. As you are driving to your midday appointment, awaiting your next client's arrival, or just have a few free minutes, take the time to record your magical moments that occurred throughout the day or one you remember in your life.

If you want to have a written version of your recorded magical moment, it is really easy. Once I have a few recorded, I email them to a transcriber who transcribes them and then sends the file back to me. There are many online transcribing services that can do this relatively inexpensively. Shortly thereafter, you will receive a written version of those magical moments you sent off. These are easily preserved and allow you the occasion to create lasting memories in your life – a few minutes at a time.

Doctor's Appointment – *A Son Grows Up*

It's 3:30 p.m. and I am waiting for Justin, my teenage son, to finish his first doctor's appointment on his own. It caught me a bit off guard when he said to me, "Mom, I don't need you to come in with me. I am old enough to go by myself." After my initial surprise, I felt an unfamiliar lump in my throat realizing that my boy had grown into a man. When did that happen? I paused to reflect on that moment and then walked into the medical office corridor. I turned on the voice-recording app on my phone.

> *It's twenty-four years ago; time sure passes quickly. We have visited the kindergarten and all the papers are complete to start elementary school. I can't believe my baby boy is already going to school. It was just a moment ago that I rocked him to sleep in his soft blue pajamas with his little bear. The last thing we need to do before school starts is get his immunization shots at the doctor's office. I sit in the waiting room, watching him play with the toys and look at the books in the children's area. The nurse calls us in. I take his hand and we walk to the private room. The nurse checks his height and weight and pats him on the back. The doctor comes in, looks him over, and tells him he is growing up to be such a big boy. Justin smiles proudly and stands a little taller. Then the nurse comes in with a tray of syringes. I know what is coming but Justin doesn't. The doctor lifts him onto the table and lifts up Justin's shirtsleeve. After a swipe of alcohol, he inserts the first needle and we all immediately hear the familiar sounds of a child's wail throughout the office. After several attempts, we finally, as a team, hold Justin for the other two shots. Once we finished, Justin bolted from the room and went directly to*

the center of the office and yelled from the top of his lungs, "I will never come to the doctor's again. I don't like any of you, and I will never, never, never come here again!"

I turn off the recording and walk back into the waiting room to find Justin patiently waiting for me. "All done, Justin?"

He replies, "Yes, I just need to come back in a week for a shot. I can drive myself." I smile at him and we walk silently to the car. When I arrive home, I download my recording and email it to Chili, the transcriber I use. Just a few days later, I open my email to find the story typed and ready to add into my magical moments journal.

I take every moment I can to add to my collection of magical moments. Have you ever had a fleeting memory that put a smile on your face, and then in a flash it was gone? The point is, you don't have to lose those moments. Now you can capture them anywhere, at any time. Remember, magical moments come and go in an instant. Any way to preserve these moments will pay back enormous dividends over the course of your life and will help to build your legacy. It's like making a deposit into the bank of your life, but the dividends and benefits will last a lifetime.

REFLECT

- How meaningful would it be to have an audio or written version of these magical moments for your children, your grandchildren, or even for yourself to remember the gifts in your life?
- What would have to happen for you to press "record" today and capture your first one?

Let the Music Move You

A friend is someone who knows the song in your heart and can sing it back to you when you have forgotten the words.
– Unknown

Hank Williams Sr. said, "A song ain't nothin' in the world but a story just wrote with music to it." Music is an amazing way to bring us back to the magic in our past or propel us forward to our visions of the future. Music can evoke a whole host of past magical moments with friends, family, and even those sacred moments on our own. My friend Carolyn created a song list she calls her "morning jams." Each morning she wakes up to her morning jams and those songs set the tone for her day on the right note.

How many times have you been driving and a song comes on the radio that takes you back to a special time in your life? Music is such a powerful force for many of us. We can listen to a song and immediately be transported to a moment in our past filled with a wide range of emotions and memories. Indeed, the sense of hearing can be one of our most dominant senses. Hearing a song can be a powerful trigger to our memory and is just one more way to help us capture our magical moments.

Morning Jams – Carolyn and Gina's Great Adventures

> *It was early one morning, and I woke up to my friend Carolyn boppin' to the beat of some upbeat joyful music. We had both worked long hours at a personal development program and wanted to start our day with the right energy and in a positive state. I couldn't help but wake up, grin, and move my body to the music.*

"It's my morning jams!" she said. "I wake up each morning to this music, and it sets my great mood and starts me off on the right foot."

Carolyn's morning jams were one of the many things that began a lifelong friendship. She is more than family to me; she is my soul sister. We have drifted apart as our lives have taken different turns. But I still have those morning jams on a playlist. When I press play and hear that music, a flood of memories and magical moments flows through my mind and I can't help but smile. That music opens such a special place in my mind...

Racing jet skis in the Caribbean – she loves to go fast. Working eight days straight with little sleep – we woke up laughing uncontrollably and both knew what for! Match.com dates – people really did post those messages! Being stood up on both of our blind dates one evening – we ended up dancing and on the beach in La Jolla. Surfing lessons – Nick saved our lives when we were in over our heads, really! My bags getting stolen from our car in Hawaii – Carolyn saved the wedding. The surf instructor saying "I don't like engineers and lawyers" – he didn't know Carolyn was an engineer and I was a lawyer. Volleyball at the beach, birthday parties, roommates with piles of stuff everywhere, baking with my kids, "Don't tempt me," Gabi and Gilbert at Jack's at the same time, "Send the 5-carat ring and I'll meet you at the Elvis Chapel in Vegas," gambling, Hawaii, that dress looks like it's from a Hofbrau Haus, "Of course you can run this race on the beach," Game on!, ordering the plus-one garden salad instead of the full filet mignon meal, "Could you jump off that boat and swim to shore?," hiking and singing "Rise and shine...," being "surfer chicks," I've got tickets!, "Who are the two elves?," marzipan people on my wedding cake, and so much more....

Carolyn's inspiration in my life has been a blessing. Magical moments – yes, we certainly had our share. The laughter, the tears, the joy, the sadness, the challenge, and all the colors of the rainbow graced the stories of our friendship. Just taking the time to remember those magical moments now, I feel a tear in one eye and a smile in the other. The power of true friendship and the gift of taking a moment to remember are amazing!

Carolyn – As that inspiring song reminds us, "God bless the broken road that led me straight to you."

Many artists and musicians communicate their magical moments and stories through music. Most songs are stories communicated through music. The artistry of a talented musician not only tells a story but also captures the emotion that brings a story to life. Thus, music is truly a passionate and creative manner by which to relay your magical moments to others; it also creates a bountiful and nourishing backdrop for more magical moments to be created.

Music helps to open the door to the heart and soul. The unconscious inspiration in music triggers and resonates at a high level, which can promote an outpouring of emotions and memories of special times. To capture more magical moments, begin by hitting play on the soundtrack of your life.

REFLECT

- What songs can you remember that represent a magical time in your life?
- When was the last time you listened to one of those songs?
- What songs would motivate and empower you for your future?
- Can you think of those songs now?
- What songs would you put in your "Morning Jams" and "Inspiration" playlists?

A Special Place

Similar to the music trigger, magical moments often correspond with scenery. As you position yourself in beautiful and inspiring places, you will find the occurrence of more magical moments. Think about some of the happiest moments in your life. I bet they occurred with loved ones at the beach, or in the mountains, or maybe in a foreign country on a blissful vacation. Here is an example of a journal entry I made while traveling in Italy:

Inside the Book's Cover – *A Traveler's Library of Journeys*

I am walking on the cobblestone streets in Florence, Italy. I have a mission on this day to find just the right book. It's getting late and the evening shadows are dancing on the streets. I pause at the window of a well-kept but aging store with a weathered Italian man inside. As I enter, I feel like I am standing in a slice of history. You rarely see books like these. The bindings are trimmed in such beautiful designs. Some have deep rich leather bindings with gold gilded pages. Others are deep reds, browns, and tans with ornate detail. You just don't see this level of craftsmanship in modern books. The gentleman there is the owner of the shop and I explain what I want.

"Each time I travel, I love wandering the streets of a city in search of a book that reflects the spirit and culture from that special place. At the end of my trip I open the book, and inside the cover I write some of the magical moments from my trip – phrases, chance encounters with people, funny moments with family and friends, my thoughts about my life, joyful and challenging times, and things that really can't be captured in just photos. My library at home is filled with these books, each holding many of my life's magical moments."

The bookshop owner smiles, and in a mixture of Italian and English we search the store together. From past experience, I know that the right book will appear. We find a beautiful book series written in Italian called Istorie Fiorentine. This is perfect! He wraps each book in tissue paper and carefully ties them up with some dusty string. He hands them over to me as if he is presenting me with a sacred treasure. His pride in his shop and his books still resonates within those books. I leave there completely satisfied that this trip's books are safe and secure and ready to be filled with the magical moments from this adventure.

Traveling to new places and experiencing different cultures and environments will open the door for magical moments to come in. We focus enormous time and energy on our careers, but it is imperative to schedule time to simply get away. An annual vacation, time off with your family, even a quick trip to the beach or mountains when the workload is light will pay great dividends in your ability to experience magical moments. This traveler uses antique books to record memories from her journeys. I have found these treasures in so many unique places, and just those memories make me happy!

And when you do travel, make sure you bring along your camera and a journal so that when time permits you can step back, reflect on your time away from it all, and put pen to paper to capture the magical moments.

REFLECT

- Can you remember the last time you took time away from your daily routine to experience another place?
- Were you with friends or family or spending sacred time alone?
- What was magical during that time? The people you met? The food you ate? The sounds of silence? Nature? Fun outside your daily life?

- What specifically made that trip worthwhile?
- When is the next time you have scheduled a break from your normal daily life?

A Picture Is Worth a Thousand Words

So many magical moments are captured not just with your memory, but also with your camera or other recording device. Over the years I have found it helpful to take lots of pictures and once per month sit down with these pictures and review them. I took the picture because something about the scene or the people or even the moment struck a chord in my soul. So it is extremely possible that those pictures are simply visual representations of magical moments.

But don't rely solely on your camera or video recorder. The most powerful tool you have at your disposal is your mind. When you find yourself in a magical moment, take a deep breath and survey the picture in front of you. Look it over and then close your eyes. Open them again and visualize the serenity you are experiencing. Repeat this for a few minutes until you can accurately capture the image with your eyes closed. This exercise will help you to compartmentalize the image and remember the beauty in front of your eyes. Take time often to re-visualize this moment and record it to memory. By doing so, you will always have magical moments within your mind's reach, allowing you to use them as valuable tools to find peace and locate happiness when life becomes hectic and stressful.

REFLECT

- When was the last time you looked at your family photo albums?
- When have you set aside time to really pause and remember the magic in each of those fleeting life moments?

- Is it possible for you to set aside a few moments this week to appreciate and enjoy just a few of those pictures to find the magical moment in each of them?

Same Time Next Year

The list of ways to capture magical moments is endless. Throughout this chapter we have given you some ideas, and you can also take time to find your own ways to capture these exciting and endless opportunities. We all live different lives, and there may be facets of your life that lend themselves to a different manner by which to capture these moments.

Some years I write in my journal. Other years I videotape my magical moments. Sometimes I just record my thoughts from the past. In recent years I have enlisted my children's help to create a "year in review" iMovie that we enjoy on New Year's Eve as a family. In our lives, hours pass, days pass, months pass, and then years pass. Can you imagine a moment in your life where you open a box to find years of memories in one place? You find your writing from December 31, 2000, and smile, reflecting on your life then and now. You find the video from 1985 and a tear falls from your eye as you remember that was the last year you spent time with your loving father. You find a recording from 1984 when your first son was born, and you hear his baby gurgles and your own voice singing to him.

On December 31 of each year I have a ritual I have done for years – I go to the beach or the lake and sit with a journal enjoying the waves and the gentle dialogue between surf and sand. I ask myself, "What has to happen this next year so that I can say 'WOW, that was the best year of my life?'" For me, it's often having special sacred magical moments with my family, friends, and new people in my life.

By the Water's Edge – *A New Year's Tradition*

It's December 31, 2010, and I am sitting by myself at the snowy edge of Big Bear Lake. Most of the lake is frozen, and even though the sun is shining, it is really cold. I wrap myself in my winter jacket and start to write.

This year, I married the true love of my life, Greg. I am not sure if he really knows the gift he is in my life and the magic we share together. Standing on the shores of the beach in Hawaii, feeling the warm sand in my toes, and then paddling out on our surfboards to declare our never-ending love for each other was one of the most profound moments in my life.

This is just one example of how I take time to reflect on my magical moments over the year past. But don't wait until the last day of the calendar year to reflect. On some level, reflection should occur on a daily basis. Even if it is just for a few moments before you go to bed, or right when you awaken, take time each day, each week, each month, and each year to evaluate, identify, and then celebrate the occurrences in your life that have truly influenced you.

Capturing magical moments is crucial. Many times the magic grows as the moment is celebrated and reminisced. They start as small seeds, but each time they are repeated or evoked, they begin to sprout up and grow with meaning and significance. Find time to capture these magical moments in your own special way. There is no right or wrong answer, only action or inaction. So for purposes of capturing magical moments, just schedule the time to act.

As we move ahead, we will discuss the different segments of your life that create the most magical of moments. Time with your family, friends, and loved ones, time alone, time in nature, time serving the greater good, and living a life destined to create a lasting legacy will all invite an amazing and diverse array of magical moments into your life.

Together, we will delve into each of these important parts of your life and the vital steps you can take now to remember and create magical moments for the rest of your life.

5

Magical Moments within Families

Love your family. Spend time together.
Be kind, and serve one another.
Make no room for regrets.
Tomorrow is not promised to anyone and today is short.

– Author Unknown

In the previous chapter we outlined some inspirational ways to capture magical moments. These should be used as the traditional, big ideas that can be applied to any and every situation. But the remainder of this book will shift to identifying the most magical of magical moments and then offering you specific and detailed ways to optimize the magic in each of these areas of your life. With that in mind, the most likely place to start is with your family.

The Oxford Dictionary defines a family as "a group consisting of parents and children living together in the same household." Now, that is a traditional definition of the word. But for our purposes, let's expand this concept. A family is more than just people related by blood. A family is a group of people that are connected and care for one another. They may live together, work together, or just simply spend time together. It is not defined by the amount of time but rather by the quality of time. Families care about one another at a very high level. They look forward to seeing one another, sharing stories, experiencing moments, and exchanging love and emotions. Families are everywhere and transcend generations, sex, economic status, regions, background, and upbringing. A family is not something you can define; it is something you feel. When you care and love another, he or she is your family.

So, as we continue along together on our journey of creating magical moments, remember that your family is a special group of people connected by love and emotion. But also remember that everyone has a different definition of family. There is no "acceptable" definition in any dictionary to define family. It is a personal and special dynamic that you get to define yourself.

Traditions

If you ask one of our children to share a magical moment, you will hear the familiar sigh of a child who knows a family tradition like they know their home. They know it's a time to pause, reflect, and recall an event in their lives that was meaningful to them. This continues to be one of the many ways we share our lives with each other, learn what is important to each of us, and cherish life with loved ones and those who spend time with us.

Magical moments in families happen every day. Unfortunately, most families are so busy that they rarely take notice. In the circle of life, it is inevitable that when one thing ends, another begins. That is life. Yet, as parents, in our zeal to celebrate and lift our kids into their next accomplishment and stage of life, we forget to take a moment to be grateful for the times that signify an end of an era. These "last times" are their transition and turning point into the next phase of their lives – the last time they crawled, climbed on your lap, asked you to tuck them in and so many more. It is our responsibility to stop to take the time to disconnect ourselves and our families from modern life so we can collectively smell the roses in real life.

REFLECT

- Can you remember the last time you tucked your child in at night? Kissed them goodnight?
- Can you remember the last time you told your child you loved them?
- What "last times" are about to happen in their life?
- Can you capture those magical moments?

Children are amazing at capturing and experiencing the moment. Just watch the joy in a group of children playing. They know how to live in the moment and soak up every minute of those magical moments. As we get older, we seem to be caught up more in the "to-do list" and getting things done each day. We tend to lose our spontaneity and carefree spirit to continually focus on the next thing to do. When was the "last time" you lived in the moment?

His Last Night at Home – *Justin's Story*

> *My oldest son, Justin, is thirty. One of the things I remember most*
> *was the joy I would feel in his accomplishments. I remember his*
> *first play, his passion for science, his first date, his senior prom,*
> *his sneaking out of the house while a teenager, and especially his*
> *first night away at college.*
>
> *I remember going to the store in Boston and buying him all the*
> *things he would need in his dorm room at Boston University. As*
> *his mom, I of course didn't want him to go without anything so I*
> *really stocked his room full. As I left him that day, I cried all the*
> *way to the airport realizing that he had lived his last day at home.*
> *Did I take a moment to cherish that day? To celebrate the eigh-*
> *teen years he lived under my roof? To embrace that last time that*
> *really was a bridge to his adulthood? I realized in my zealousness*
> *to move my child ahead through life, that for eighteen years I had*
> *celebrated his accomplishments, his transitions to getting older,*
> *his first times for so many things, that I didn't take the time to*
> *cherish those last times that were the real magic in his life.*

From childhood to adulthood, there is a bridge our children cross over
to their own lives. We never really know when it happens but it does,
and celebrating and capturing the magical moments will help you
appreciate and give meaning to that circle of life. Thus, it is time to
begin building traditions – now. Small traditions turn into large ones at
an exciting pace. For example, think about the parents who implement
a family rule that everyone eats dinner together without cell phones or
other technology. The simple act of sharing a meal can lead to an amazing array of magical moments. But even if they don't, the worst-case
scenario is that you make time and find a moment to speak to your
husband or wife to catch up on your child's experiences and life as it
happens. No matter what, start the small traditions now to create a habit
of these behaviors. Once you do that, you will begin to impact your
family and its development at an extremely high level.

How to Create and Capture Magical Moments within Families

At Meals…

There are numerous opportunities to create magical moments with your family. And as mentioned above, it can start with something as small as sharing a meal together. At each breakfast, lunch, or dinner, ask everyone at the table to share a magical moment. Remember, a magical moment can be anything; it can be something that occurred at school or at work, an experience they had on the bus, or even an event they attended over the weekend. As my children grew older, I could see that their lives and experiences were growing and their magical moments reflected their maturity into adulthood.

Creating a tradition with your family is powerful in the life of a child. If you ask children to recall their childhood, many will recall the things that their families did over and over again. This conditioning creates a powerful element in the life stories, the magical moments, and the history of a child.

You can create a tradition of sharing magical moments at your dinner table. You can share each night, at Sunday dinners, or even on holidays. The point is that your children will grow up to understand that sharing their moments in life with their family is an important part of their family history. They will start focusing on moments and mentally taking note that this or that event will be great to share as a magical moment.

You can learn so much about other people by listening to their magical moments. You may sometimes be surprised to hear what others believe is magical. In those moments you discover what people hold as important, what they value in life, and what is most memorable to them. I have found that this is especially true with our children. When we share magical moments at our dinner table, I learn so much about my children and how their lives are developing.

North End of Boston – A College Visit

One of my favorite magical moments was my first visit to my son's college when he attended Boston University. It was a cold winter evening in Boston. I arrived at my son's apartment to greet all seven of his friends that I was taking to dinner—hungry college boys who loved when parents came to visit. It meant a delicious dinner out, which always beat the dorm food. We arrived at this old-school Italian restaurant in the North End of Boston. After we settled in at our table, I raised my glass to toast the boys, and of course I asked if I could share a family tradition that night. I saw my son visibly roll his eyes, as he knew what was coming. I learned so much about his friends that night. One of them shared that he was training to go into the air force. One shared a story about being a die-hard Red Sox fan and what that meant to him. Another shared how much he enjoyed my son's healthy cooking since he was raised on meat and potatoes every night.

Even more magical to me was my next visit when one of my son's friends told me that he went home for the holidays and started the magical moments tradition with his family. He said he had a large family and most dinners were loud and full of arguments and banter. He said it was unbelievable. Everyone shared. They were even quiet and respectful during those shares—unbelievable! They truly loved hearing those magical moments from each other. He said they learned more about each other in that one meal than they had in years.

Can We Tell Magical Moments? – Dave, Dawnie, and Henry's Story

We had been telling magical moments around the dinner table with friends for years at events (birthdays, Thanksgiving, "family" meals as we call them with our close friends), sharing something personal with everyone, but never at home. There were only two of us at the dinner table, and to be frank, when we were at a large gathering my husband, Dave, and I often felt a sense of mild panic that we wouldn't be able to come up with a magical moment and something meaningful or witty to share.

That changed once our son Henry arrived. He began to experience the fun of magical moments when we were at large gatherings before he was able to talk. Then finally when he was about two and a half, we were at a birthday meal with around twelve people at the table when magical moments began. Henry got so excited he started jumping up and down, desperate for his turn! He wanted the full attention of the table and shouted "My magical moment...hoop...hoop" and threw his arm in the air to show he was trying to get a basketball in the hoop.

From that day onwards, we started to talk about magical moments each evening around the dinner table, sharing something special from our day with our family. And now, aged three and a half, Henry is the one who asks every night "Can we tell magical moments?" On a recent holiday visiting his grandparents, aunty, uncle, and cousin in Australia, he got them all into the habit by initiating "let's do magical moments" and then telling each person whose turn it was next. He melted everyone's heart when he said, "My magical moment is seeing you guys."

During Holidays and Birthdays…

Holidays are a very special time for togetherness and cohesion. In fact, holidays bring together families that may otherwise not see one another during the year. Distance, scheduling, or just plain resistance can often create a gap in the ability for families to share time together. So use holidays as an excuse to reconnect and create meaningful moments. The simple yet sometimes arduous task of assembling all the members of your family in one room can seem impossible. But once you do, it can provide amazing opportunities to create magical moments.

Too Much Stuff – *Magical Moments Coupons*

> *One Christmas I realized that each year our children were given so many gifts that after the first few gifts much of the sentiment was lost in the piles of toys, clothes, gift cards, and endless "stuff." One year I decided to change this, and instead of giving massive amounts of things, I decided to give each of my children the gift of a magical moment. So I gave them a creatively designed coupon for a special time with me during the year. One year I gave my ten-year-old daughter a coupon to go to her first concert with me. We went to the Staples Center to see the High School Musical concert. We still talk about it even now when she is a teen in high school. Another year I was lucky enough to find an opportunity for my son and me to be honorary team captains for the Los Angeles Lakers. It was an amazing highlight that year to step onto the court with my son and shake Kobe Bryant's hand and share our thoughts for that evening's game. I have surprised my husband with coupons for a weekend away snowboarding and so much more. These moments continue to create so much more depth and magic in our lives than things. I am so excited to see what we will experience together this coming year.*

You can give magical moments to your family members as wedding gifts, for birthday presents, and for any special occasion. It helps us remember the value of time together rather than just the things we give each other. Always find an excuse (like a holiday or birthday) to create a magical moment.

Raising a Son – *A Single Mom's Milestones*

I raised my oldest son by myself from the time he was born. As a single parent, I worried endlessly about who would care for my son if something happened to me. I remember that each year on his birthday I would pause and take a moment to be grateful that he was another year older. My focus seemed to be more on who would care for him if something happened to me and less on the magic in the moments of his youth. Each year propelled him another year closer to adulthood. I was so grateful each time he reached another milestone in his life that I rarely paused to appreciate the last times. I never really savored the beauty of his childhood but instead focused on his crossing over each bridge to his next era and phase of life. The last time he crawled, his last soccer game, his last birthday party with balloons, the last night he had a curfew – I feel like I missed them all! Looking back now, there were so many opportunities to cherish and appreciate, and now I spend time capturing as many of those moments as I can remember.

At Bedtime…

Those special moments before you and your loved ones go to bed are truly inspiring and are riveting opportunities to create magical moments. Bedtime is a special time with families. Many families read bedtime stories and say prayers before a cozy sound sleep. This is such a magical time for families and a perfect time in a peaceful quiet place to share special moments together. It can be as easy as sharing a magical moment with your child and asking your child to share a magical moment with you. Think of all the wonderful life moments you can share with your children so they can learn more about you and you can continue to learn more about them.

The beauty of bedtime is that your children don't even need to be awake to experience a meaningful magical moment with them. For years, I would regularly walk into my children's room after they went to sleep and listen to them breathe or watch them sleep. It gave me a sense of wonderment and ease when I could watch this amazingly blissful little being slip away into his or her dreams. The younger your children are, the more special the experience can seem. Can you remember the last time you watched your newborn baby sleep and appreciated the blessing of this new soul in your life?

Sweet Dreams – *Chuck's Story*

> *Last night I walked into my eldest child's room to check up on him as I have done each night of his life when I have had the privilege of being home. Now fourteen years old and knee deep in the transition into manhood, I realized that this young man was the same blessed soulful child that blessed our lives with such an amazing torrent of love and excitement back in 2000. It was so surreal because in that moment of watching him rest, I was transported back to that first night he came home from the hospital and how excited and grateful I was to have our boy home. I remember so vividly watching his little belly move up and down with each slow, deep, cleansing breath. I recall the feeling of the calm, divine energy of rest and relaxation as I felt the presence of this new gift that was bestowed to my wife and me. I pondered what my boy might be dreaming as I observed little smiles and facial expressions. Time seemed to stand still, and I cannot recall how long I stood over him and witnessed such a simple yet humbling event. As I turned to leave his room and close his door I glanced back and spied a last look at my boy, and I caught myself feeling warm and so grateful for each and every experience I have been gifted to be a part of.*

I look forward to checking up on all my children and taking a moment to remember the love, laughter, and excitement each of them has brought to our world.

Give yourself a gift and "Remember the last time you...?"

Dinosaur Night Light and Other Bedtime Necessities – *The Lin Family Story*

We had just gotten back from the Los Angeles Kings hockey game with our two kids and had tucked them into bed around 9 p.m. They both were extremely tired from a very eventful weekend—we were too! Our three-year-old Max did his usual routine of asking for everything under the sun to be in bed with him, including five hockey pucks, his hockey stick, two very important nunnies (his blankets), an array of stuffed animals, a glass of water, and the most important thing – his Triceratops night light.

After getting Max settled and delivering his glass of water, our six-year-old daughter Emma came out from her bedroom crying because she wanted me to sleep with her. I firmly told her that she needed to sleep in her own bed like a big girl and tucked her in again. Two more times she came out, and once again I took her back to her room. The revolving bedroom doors of parents with little kids are alive and active at our house each night!

The last time that Emma got out of bed, she just stood at her doorway crying about the bad thought (dream) she had that all the bad dreams were in her closet and would come out to get her when she closed her eyes. I went to her again and reassured her that all was well and she was safe. I returned to my husband, Felix, in the living room, while we awaited the hopeful silence.

The next thing we heard was Max getting out of his bed and walking down the hall. Just as we were getting up AGAIN to make another trip down the hall to Max's room, we heard Max talking to Emma as he gave her his favorite Triceratops night-light to scare away her bad dreams.

In that magical moment, Felix and I sighed and welled up knowing that we were raising children who were growing up to be loving, caring individuals, and when the time comes they will love and protect each other despite their own fears.

Of course, Emma – age six – told her brother, "I don't want it!" But it's a start...

In Your Home...

They say your home is where your heart is. Even more exciting is the notion that your home is where all your hearts are. Your home is a place of solace, comfort, and happiness. We have a beautiful sign in our home that says: "Home is where your story begins." I often look at that sign and ask myself, what is really "home"? How many homes have I had so far in this lifetime? Can I remember the last time in each of those homes? Or is the memory of my life's experiences in those places enough?

Remember that your home is the special place where you share memories and magical moments. It does not have to be a mansion or be filled with the most lavish "things." What matters is that it is supported and protected with love and respect. Houses change, families move on. But love and connectivity are the commonality that can easily be moved to any new abode.

Moving Out! – *Vicki's Story*

In the last two or three years we've had a couple of financial challenges. In January of last year negotiations between us and our principal financiers went from average to really bad, leading them to appoint receivers on a couple of our companies and on most of our properties. Unfortunately one of these properties was our own home that we'd built about five years previously. Whilst it was never going to be our final home, we were pretty happy living there. So preparing for the day we had to leave required lots of focus.

The thing is, with the right attitude you can turn any bad situation into a good or great one, and I took this as an opportunity to get rid of lots of stuff! It was really good to empty out cupboards, drawers, and boxes—not only finding things that were no longer required, but also lots of memories and souvenirs from various travels over the years. I especially loved finding things I had thought were gone for good! It also felt really good to be able to give away stuff I no longer needed to someone who had a use for it, be it a friend, family member, or a charity.

We made the decision on when to move out and decided to do it on our own terms before we were officially "asked to leave." One of my favorite places in the house was our home theatre, and we'd had many, many great nights there watching movies, favorite shows, and of course lots of sporting events. (It was quite a common event for the two of us to spend all night in the "dungeon" as a friend had once labeled it!)

On our last night before we had the "removalists" coming to collect everything, we watched Avatar – a movie I had seen when it was at the cinema, but not since. It was wonderful to be able to appreciate the fabulous setup that we had, both with the sound and vision, for the last time.

One of the funny things is that sometimes the difference between a house and a home is you, your memories, and what you have in the place, and I couldn't believe it, but once we'd taken everything out and done a final tidy up, the place became a house again, and

even my favorite room, the home theatre, was just a room. I'm
grateful for the memories we were able to create in that house,
and I am grateful for new ones that we have created each and
every day since.

In Your Memories...

Magical moments should not only be shared but also remembered.
Some of the most special parts of a family dynamic are the wonderful
ways in which families take the time to remember these moments. As
you grow your family, choose either a parent or an older child and
appoint that person with the responsibility of collecting these magical
moments. This can be done through photographs, videos, diaries, note-
books, or audio recordings. There are many tools and resources out
there to truly collect these memories, so you should never be at a loss.
Think about the exciting opportunity to look back years from now and
enjoy these moments again.

Most families have family albums to share treasured memories. Consider starting albums and storybooks of your family's magical moments
in life. Capturing and documenting the magical moments you share can
transform a photo album of a vacation. There are so many moments in
life, from the time a couple falls in love and even from the time a child
is born, that are never heard by family members. There are so many
resources for saving these memories—a quick recording on a cell
phone, a short video, in a brief writing, on a note in your computer, or
even on a napkin in a restaurant. There are so many easy ways to capture them!

Chance Encounters – *Kevin and Patti's Love Story*

Ever have a brief chance meeting with someone who leaves you
wondering "what if"?

– Alexia Chianis

Patti: This is the story of how two lives were changed in a night, a magical moment that grew from a chance encounter…

I was living in West Hollywood and it was a Friday night. I told my friend I was NOT going out that night, but she insisted that I come down to Hermosa Beach with her for a quiet "beach bar" night and said she would be by to get me in fifteen minutes. I had no idea that I would meet my future husband that very night.

But there he was…on the patio at Patrick Malloy's. I knew I wanted to talk to him. Something about his energy and the way he glanced my way made the butterflies in my stomach come alive! I'll never forget that moment…the magical moment that made me believe in the possibility of love and wonder; it was a moment I never thought I could feel for myself, for I had only heard descriptions of others' experiences.

That moment was just about ten years ago. And I still feel the butterflies even as I come home from the grocery store and see his truck parked in the driveway.

I am truly blessed and will be forever grateful for the magical moment my eyes met his. I love you, Kevin. Thank you for living this life with me. I can't wait to make so many more magical moments with you.

Kevin: Sometimes magical moments hold and deepen their power with time. What may seem like any other day can have synchronistic veins that become apparent, steadily and gradually, evolving into an emotion or connection that could never have been comprehended, let alone imagined. In 2002, I was heading down to the pier for some late summer fun and folly that I had been in the business of for most of that season. It was the end of a beautiful month and a brilliant day; the sun was slowly slipping past the sea, and the clouds were reflecting a brilliant purplish orange glow that only God or Van Gogh could create.

She walked past me once and then again. I smiled, and as she walked past again my roommate and a friend struck up a conversation with her. I don't remember much about what was said other than some rude comments from my roommate and the fact that my friend was hitting on her, but I felt a warmth spread over me that made me pause and turn inward. We shook hands, and as I looked in her eyes I felt the stirrings of something I had never felt and could not articulate. She had friends inside and was down at the beach visiting from Hollywood and had to move on. We were locals just kicking it on the pier putting on airs and working on being cool. She left to head up the Avenue to another club. When she had left I was still tingling; something unexplained was in the air. My friend turned and said, "She likes you, man, go get her," and there it was. Those words shot through me, and I headed up the hill and stood in the doorway as she walked out of the ladies' room and up to me.

The rest of the evening, the rest of my life ever since, has been full of spirit and magic and love. A magical moment that gains momentum and builds as I fall in love with Patti over and over again with each passing day…

The Winning Poem – *A Love Competition*

I had just recently met a wonderful man and then I had to leave the country for work. I was across the ocean in Australia. For me, there is magic in that feeling of falling in love. The excitement of being with someone special, the anticipation and butterflies in your stomach when you know you will be with them, the sheer joy of their company, and the longing for him or her when you are not together—the magic of love.

While I was working at that event overseas, we exchanged a few emails. He would write his during the day while I was asleep in Australia, and I would wake up to his email each morning and send him one in return. Sheer delight.

My friend Buzz was working with me at the event, and she had just met a new love in her life. We were sharing our love stories and laughed and smiled a lot together. After a few days of sharing text messages and emails, we decided on a friendly competition for who would receive the best message from their new love. One of the rules was that you could not tell your man about the game – the message had to come naturally...

After a few days of exchanging messages, Buzz brought her phone to me and declared, "I win!"

She had just received a text message that said "I am coming to take what is mine!" and she found out he was traveling across Australia just to be with her.

Wow – hard to beat that... I thought she was the winner...

Then on the last day of our event, and the last day of our contest, I woke up to see this email in my inbox—one of the most magical moments in my life.

"Good afternoon to you my shining star...you'll see in a minute I am no poet, but I need to address my feelings as I sit here tonight.

Imagining the distant paths of souls as they travel the road of life.

Two wandering lives meet, destinies intertwined, past experiences now forgotten,

Like a sail caught by a gust of wind, my soul has been moved in a direction unforeseen

Such a short time ago...

I see in you a flame, an image so warm, so beautiful, so full of inspiration.

This flame, this light, has captivated my soul, has allowed my mind to set itself in safe harbor.

Like a flame, I am attracted to its offerings, its mysteries, its passions, and the protection it brings from foreign forces.

To me you are my flame, shining brightly across the sea as if a star twinkling magnificently in the night sky.

I gaze upon your light, knowing that each night your warmth will return, forever keeping my soul in safe harbor."

Suffice it to say, I emailed it to the front desk and asked them to print it out. Then I ran down to pick it up so I wouldn't be late for our team meeting. I dropped the printed email in front of Buzz and declared myself "Winner!"

Truly, Buzz and I were both winners. We had such magical moments together sharing our dreams of love and happiness.

For me, I had another magical moment when I married this man on July 3, 2010, and he remains my true love and sheer magic in my life.

This isn't exact math. But it is about taking the time and exerting the effort to capture these memories, so schedule the time to record these moments as they occur. Enlist the help of your family; they will truly embrace the occasion to become CMMOs (Chief Magical Moment Officers).

As Children Grow…

Children are amazing at capturing and experiencing the moment. So take the time to enjoy the moments as your children grow. They are so special and change at a rapid pace.

The Last Time I Tripped – *Debz's Story*

When my son Stephen was a teenager I used to get upset every time I tripped over his size fourteen shoes. It was his habit to walk in the door, kick off his shoes, and leave them conveniently placed so anyone who had a mind to could trip over them. The step down from the entry into the living room made this especially hazardous.

The number of times I pleaded, cajoled, or scolded to get him to do something different ranks in the hundreds or even thousands. Logical suggestions of what he could do differently, that would be almost as easy, had zero impact. His shoes were still there EVERY DAY. Even though I knew they would be, I still managed to trip over them from time to time.

One fall afternoon I arrived home from work early, walked in the door, looked at my husband, and started sobbing uncontrollably. My husband freaked out, not knowing what the heck was wrong with me.

When I could finally catch my breath in between the blubbering, I said, "I didn't trip. His shoes aren't here. He's gone and he's not coming home again. I miss him!" Stephen had left for college a few weeks earlier.

As much as I thought I was ready for him to be grown up and on to a life of his own, that day it sank in. I'd tripped over his shoes for the last time. Our life as a family had changed and the shoes showed me how. Stephen would never live at home again. After college he traveled, then married, and now has a family of his own. I hope he's tripping over shoes and will one day realize what a blessing that truly is.

Mummy, Please Pick Me Up – *Ashley's Story*

Grace will be five on Monday, and somehow the small steps between my current four-year-old preschooler and my soon-to-be five-year-old kindergartener seem like a vast chasm between two different lands – the land of infinite cuddles, kisses, hugs, I love yous, and the sweet peal of mirth that is the sacred bookmark of this precious age...and the land of seemingly instant independence where this sweet child of mine is suddenly making her bed, cleaning her room, taking her plates to the sink without being asked, and saying things like "I can do it by myself."

When Grace was about three and a half, an old back injury of mine flared up and carrying my preschooler became a painful and not particularly intelligent endeavor. At the same time, she suddenly wanted to be picked up ALL THE TIME. "My legs are tired" became the phrase du jour – from the kitchen to her bedroom, from the driveway to the front door, from the car park to the shop thirty feet away – we seemed to suddenly stumble upon an invisible leg zapper that kicked in after about ten steps, and which reduced my perfectly mobile and usually docile three-year-old to an unyielding and immovable force of gravity.

"Please carry me," she would plead.

"Grace, darling, I would love to carry you, but you are too big for me to carry now because my back is hurt," I would respond.

"Pleeeeeeeeeze?"

"Grace, you are too big to carry, and it hurts my back too much."

"But my legs hurt."

"Grace, I just told you – you are too big to carry, and it hurts my back."

"But pleeeeeeze?"

"Grace, please stop asking me to carry you. The answer is no."

And so on and so forth, ad infinitum, in the eternal looping dialogue that only a child can sustain. We seemed to have this conversation at least four times a day. Sometimes I would give in, but most of the time I maintained my position and Grace would ultimately – usually after a pint-sized royal meltdown – stomp up beside me with her little arms folded angrily across her chest and her little face all bunched up in miniature fury accompanied by a sparse, smattering of spillover tears.

This scene played out over and over again for months – it felt like forever – until one day I realized she had stopped asking and I didn't even know when that had happened.

Grace has just returned from the UK, where she spent two weeks visiting her grandparents with her father. For the two weeks she was gone, I roamed back and forth across my house like a restless caged lioness, waiting for my cub to come home. I kept looking in her bedroom, as if she might suddenly materialize from space – willing her to be beamed up from Buckingham Palace – and sleeping with her plush bunny rabbit cradled to my chest through the night to have something of hers close to me. I missed her with such fierce longing and intensity that sometimes I just wanted to kneel down and wail.

Finally, after two endless weeks, my little girl came home, and when I saw her I ran to her and swooped her up in my arms whooping with delight. I just wanted to smother her with love and kisses and never let her go again. She giggled and laughed and then abruptly, in a calm and quiet voice, said, "Mummy, please put me down." I looked at her with surprise but did as she asked and reluctantly put her down. Then I knelt beside her with my hands on her arms and asked, "Grace, what's the matter, sweetheart?"

She took a step in toward me and tenderly stroked my cheek as she fixed her wide blue eyes on mine with such total and unadulterated love. "Mummy," she said, "I'm too big for you to carry, and it hurts your back too much."

Had I so much as even contemplated what the pain of that gentle and compassionate rebuff might feel like in all those times she had pleaded with me to carry her, I would have gladly suffered a broken back to hold my daughter in my arms every time she asked, for as long as she wanted.

I could feel tears welling up in my eyes as she continued to stroke my cheek, and I hugged her close to me so she wouldn't see that a part of me had just ruptured.

Later that day we went to the shops, and I must confess that I deliberately parked in the farthest possible space and then proceeded to take her from one end of the mall to the other, running errands (that truly did need to be done).

Eventually she said, "Mummy, can we sit down for a little while? My legs are a tiny bit tired."

"Gracie," I responded, "would it be okay if I carried you? My back's better now, and no matter how big you get, you will always be my little girl."

She looked at me with those amazing blue eyes of hers and furrowed her little brow in concern and asked, "Are you sure, Mummy?"

"I am absolutely positive, my darling," I answered, with barely contained delight.

"Okay," she said tentatively, "but just for a little bit, and then I'll walk again so you don't have to carry me."

"Okay," I said, hoping she would let me carry her all the way back to the car.

I picked her up and cradled her to my chest, breathing in her wonder and her innocence and her trust, inhaling her childlike scent and brushing her cheek against mine, savoring the moment and finally appreciating the true sacredness of this fleeting time.

We're having Grace's fifth birthday party tomorrow, and I've decided that I might park the car a few blocks away from the venue. In fact, I think I'm going to make a habit of parking the car just that bit farther away, just in case Grace's legs get tired and she might agree to let me carry her.

In case you haven't already experienced it, children grow up at a lightning pace. Before you know it, your little toddler turns into a beautiful young adult. Even quicker, she will be off to college. But the magical moments can live on forever. That is, if you allow them to.

In life, there is a last time for everything. From birth to death, and especially in all the beautiful transitions as a child crosses over that magical bridge to the next phase of their life, never to return to the last phase. From infancy, to childhood, to adolescence, to adulthood, to old age, children grow into adults.

In the circle of life, it is inevitable that when one thing ends another begins. That is life. As parents, let's take a moment to be grateful for those life transitions in every stage of life—and celebrate the magical moments!

Life rarely gives us second chances, and it seems it is only when we believe we have lost our chance that we really appreciate the opportunity to have it in the first place.

I am John Smith – *The Blue Helmet Story*

Finding the picture in a box—no time for photo albums, my schedule is too busy!

This picture doesn't truly capture the magic in all the moments with that helmet when my son was a toddler.

Someone might find this picture and say, "Look how cute Oliver looks in that helmet." That just wouldn't do justice to the many magical moments that helmet represents.

We had returned from a family tour of the Hoover Dam where they gave us these blue safety helmets to wear during the tour. When we arrived home, my youngest son, Oliver, had just finished watching Pocahontas for the hundredth time. When he saw the helmet, he ran to me with such an astonished and excited gasp. He took the helmet and immediately put it on his head and declared, "Mommy, you call me John Smif and you are Pocahontas."

I replied, "Oliver, what are you talking about?"

"Mommy, I am not Oliver, I am John Smif! Like in the movie Pocahontas!" He meant John Smith, but the "th" would always come out as an "f."

This was Oliver's identity for over a year. When he first started wearing the helmet, we had to explain to him that he couldn't wear it to nursery school. That was as far as we got. When he woke up, he rolled over in his little toddler bed to lift his John Smith helmet onto his head, and from the time he came home from school to when he went to bed, the helmet was planted firmly on his head. Occasionally we got it off for a bath!

Then there were the times we lost it – oh, Oliver's tears, his upset, the inflection of power and courage in his voice when he was "John Smif," and his declaration that he "needed it." Frankly, after so long seeing it on him, he didn't look right without it. Then there was a last time he wore that helmet. I couldn't tell you when that was, but there was a last time. The blue helmet sits now on his bedroom closet shelf.

Now I sit in the college bleachers cheering on my six-foot-three son on his college basketball team remembering that not so long ago he was a toddler wearing his favorite John Smif helmet. I often wonder how many other last times there were in his life-time—the last time he sat in my lap, the last time I picked out his clothes, the last time he said "Will you tuck me in?" So many "last times" and so many magical memories. I'll just start with the blue helmet and move on from there to find and enjoy more!

It is an art to cherish those last times in each stage of our children's lives. These "last times" are the bridges to new eras and new stages of life. We often never really know when a last time is a last time. The celebration for our children reaching a new milestone overshadows an appreciation for their last time in the past phase of life.

Family: Where It All Begins...

As we continue discussing the exciting categories within life where we can create impactful magical moments, it makes sense that we have started with family. In life, nothing is more important or meaningful than family. And that goes double if you are so fortunate as to have brought a child into this world. There will be no greater responsibility than teaching, educating, and raising a young child. That beautiful and innocent little being will start with complete dependence on you to meet their needs. As they grow, so will your job. You will turn from a provider of milk to a provider of direction. You will stop changing diapers and start shaping character. You will trade teaching your child to walk for teaching them how to stand on their own two feet. But no matter what, you will always be a parent.

Life Flight, the Only Flight in the Air After 9/11 – *Greg's Story*

> *When does life take on a new meaning? When discovering that you are going to be a dad for the first time. That's when I thought I knew that life had taken on a new meaning. I knew deep inside that I wanted to be a great dad.*
>
> *I was committed to changing diapers, spending sleepless nights walking through the quiet house trying to get my little boy back to sleep, filled like all new dads with the dreams and anticipation of what my son would be, committed to the time it would take to make sure he developed values that would make him a decent human being. Having grown up in a family with great parents, I knew that I had a lot to live up to.*
>
> *Everyone remembers 9/11. I remember 9/13. Nothing prepared me for 9/13.*
>
> *Having spent a night in the hospital thinking that my eleven-day-old son had a bad cold, I struggled to make the effort to get to my*

classes and teach the following day. Probably the fact that I had just started a new teaching and coaching job at Mira Costa High School two weeks previous, spurred me to get out of bed, into the car, and to my classroom on time. I was in the middle of a lesson on world history when the school security guard walked in and said with a grim face that I was to go to the coach's office and call my wife immediately. No stopping, just get to the phone. When I called the hospital room, my son Cristian's mom told me that he was going to be life-flighted to Children's Hospital Los Angeles, and to get to the hospital immediately. My life stopped. Life-flighted? Children's Hospital LA? I thought he had a bad cold? He was only eleven days old!

I was told that my precious baby boy had a defect in his heart that essentially prevented the blood from moving out of the heart through the aorta. If it was not fixed, Cristian would die. Nothing prepared me for this experience. Life, something that we go through day after day – eat, work, exercise, socialize, beach, surf, family, eat, sleep. Routine. Life just "is" when you are thirty. Life had always been about family, friends, fun, and me.

On 9/13, life developed a new meaning for me. Life was now measured by the ability of a highly skilled group of helicopter flight crew, doctors, and nurses who could successfully deliver my bundle of life thirty-five miles across Los Angeles in time for him to have emergency surgery to repair his aorta.

Life had meaning. Life was no longer about me. Life meant something so deep, so valuable, emotion so deep that someone without a child might not even be able to understand. My brother once said after he and his wife, Leslie, had their daughter Caroline, "She completes me."

She completes me...now I get it. My son Cristian completes me. My source of completion flew in a yellow helicopter across LA on *that day, and he was the only civilian flying. As a result of 9/11 the airspace over LA was closed, and as I drove across the transition from the 105 Freeway to the 110 North, we saw the little yellow helicopter glide right through the landing path of LAX. No planes in the air. What a sight, one that no parent would ever forget.*

The magic of life, a new definition, was born for me on that day. Life for me meant that I was a dad, responsible for someone else, and I was there for someone else. That key process of maturation from thinking about yourself to thinking about others and their well-being. Not just empathy, but empathy and action.

I grew that day—I grew into being a father. It is in magical moments like this that we appreciate life and we all become better human beings.

There is nothing more meaningful than the gift of a child. There is nothing more important than raising that child. The opportunity to create magical moments will skyrocket. As you grow and your family expands, you will find that so much of what provides meaning to you is linked to those people you find in your home. Family is probably the most important category we will discuss because with a family, you have everything. Without a family, some people might find themselves looking for fulfillment and purpose. So always take the time to recognize the value in your family and realize that every moment you can share with them should be celebrated and captured in some form so you always have the opportunity to enjoy, appreciate, and relive them. Celebrate your family every day, and ensure that you give yourself and your family the time and energy they deserve.

Family Transitions...

The wiser mind mourns less for what age takes away
than what it leaves behind.

–William Wordsworth (1770-1850)

As the cycle of life progresses, many of us find ourselves challenged with aging family members, whether with Alzheimer's and other forms of dementia, physical limitations, or other health issues. Time marches on, and celebrating the magical moments with those we love is absolutely essential to finding the magic, joy, and value present in their lives.

Finding magical moments during those times of transition is a challenge in itself, yet it can be so very rewarding and serve as a powerful reminder and model for those around us. In her book *Creating Moments of Joy*, Jolene Brackey shares, "I have a vision, a vision that we will soon look beyond the challenges of Alzheimer's disease and focus more of our energy on creating moments of joy. When a person has short-term memory loss, his life is made up of moments. We are not able to create a perfectly wonderful day with those who have dementia, but it is absolutely attainable to create perfectly wonderful moments – moments that put smiles on their faces, a twinkle in their eyes, or trigger memories. Five minutes later, they won't remember what you did or said, but the feeling you left them with will linger."

Have you ever found yourself saying, "When I have some time, I will sit with my parents and record or video some of their memories and stories for my children"? Time is promised to no one. Why not make the time now. Actions speak louder than words.

Ginger Ale – *Kelly's Story*

On a recent flight to Houston to visit my father, I reflected on his life and our relationship. My father, Larry, was outgoing, friendly, generous, funny, and kind. He told great stories about his childhood in Kentucky where he grew up with his eight siblings. He was an entrepreneur. He was always up for an adventure and lived life to the fullest. So when Alzheimer's began to take over his mind at the early age of sixty, the father that I had always known started slipping away.

After twelve years of drugs, clinical trials, and a whole slew of therapies, it became clear it was time for him to live in an assisted-living facility. The hardest thing for me to accept was not being able to play tennis with him. We had always enjoyed a competitive game of tennis. Even after he was diagnosed, it always amazed me that he had the muscle memory to still psychically play tennis and most of the time to win. Eventually we stopped keeping score, but when asked who won, he would proudly tell people, "I beat the hell out of her!" I gave him a trophy with his name on it, and he would just grin from ear to ear when he saw it. It gave him a feeling of accomplishment and pride at a time in his life when most things left him feeling frustrated and incompetent. Playing tennis with dad was my gauge of the decline of his health and the progression of the disease.

At his new home I attended a support group and heard a great nugget of wisdom that I clung to because it really helped me find a new perspective. A wife of another Alzheimer's patient in the facility said this: "I see my husband as a glass of ginger ale that has been left out overnight. Most of the time it is flat, but every now and then a bubble of life will float to the top."

I started to look for the bubbles of life in my dad and cherish those moments instead of mourning all the things we couldn't do or say.

A bubble appeared when a choir came to perform at the home and he got up and asked me to dance with him in front of everyone. Another bubble appeared when he remembered my name and told me he loved me. Lots of bubbles floated to the top when I heard him whistle along with a song perfectly in tune. The biggest and best bubble of all came when I was snuggled up with him in bed watching repeats of The Golden Girls. I noticed the trophy sitting above the television. I asked, "Dad, do you see your trophy?" He grinned and replied, "Yeah, I beat the hell out of you!"

REFLECT

- What would have to happen for you to make time to sit down with your parents and other older family members to record some of their magical moments?
- What would have to happen for you to record some of your magical moments for your children and grandchildren?
- What are some of your most magical moments in life that you would like to share with the people you love?

6

The Importance of Friendships

Friends are the family we choose.

– Author Unknown

An article on friendship in *Psychology Today* quoted Anais Nin as saying, "Each friend represents a world in us, a world possibly not born until they arrive, and it is only by this meeting that a new world is born." Though some natural loners are happy without them, most of us depend greatly on the company of true friends. As with any relationship, friendships bring support and joy and occasionally strife.

Look back on your life and try to remember all the people who have touched your life. Who have you called a "friend"? As we grow older, friends will come and go, while others never leave our side. It is sometimes important to keep the old friends even when meeting new friends. There is an invisible bridge you cross starting from the time you meet someone to the magical moment when you cross over and become "friends." For many of us, that moment is intangible – it just happens. When the bridge is crossed into friendship, it is a magical moment and those memories can be cherished for life.

If you really want to know someone, look at his or her four closest friends. People tend to like people similar to them. Who are your closest friends? Who inspires you to be the best you can be? Who inspires you to follow your dreams, encourages you to be creative and find your passion, and pushes you to reach beyond your perceived limits? Likewise, we must also consider the alternative. Who prevents you from being all you can be? Who pulls you down? Who drains your energy?

Who appreciates you? Who criticizes you? Appreciation inspires people and creates a positive energy and environment in which to grow. When we feel those positive feelings such as love, we are energized and inspired to do and be more. Having friends in our lives who inspire, appreciate, and support us in reaching for our dreams is essential to living an inspired, fulfilling life full of magical moments. Alternatively, people who criticize rarely improve people or their situations. Yet many critical people continue to think their negative comments will change the other person. Do your friends inspire you and lift you, or do they criticize you and bring you down?

Who Are You as a Friend?

Now consider who you are as a friend. The magic in life is to give others the inspiration you seek from them. Do you hold yourself to the same standards you want from others? My father raised me to truly understand the maxim "The gift is the giving." So many magical moments result from that inspiration. As we inspire others to reach for their dreams and be their best, their reflection will inspire us to do the same. When we support others in shining their own unique light, we bring more light into our lives. The opposite is also true. When we prevent others from being their best or hold them back from their dreams, their reflection will prevent us from doing the same. When you create brilliance in someone's life, you bring more light into your life. When you create darkness in someone's life, your life becomes darker.

Who is in your life now, and whom do you want in your life in the future? Be the friend that will inspire and attract the people you want in your life. There are so many ways to inspire people. Sometimes it is merely a small gesture, sometimes more.

Who Are You? – *Advice from a Friend*

> *I was single and moved to a new town. It was a brave move since I didn't know anyone and wanted to start a new life. I remember talking to one of my lifelong friends and asking her advice on how to make new friends. She said make a list of all the qualities you want in a friend. So I spent time over the next few days writing out everything I wanted in a friend. I thought of friends from my past that inspired me, made me laugh, and that I cried with. So many magical moments flooded my mind. Just taking time to remember those memories was a gift. I finished my list and really felt like I nailed it – I wanted friends that had integrity, were fun, cared about their health, loved the outdoors, loved jazz, were respectful of my family, and the list went on. I called my friend back and shared the list, and then she gave me the best advice of all. She*

patiently listened to my list and then gently asked me, "Who do you need to be to attract those friends?" Wow, I spent so much time thinking about my ideal friend that the real question should have been, "Who am I as a friend?"

An article from *Sources of Insight* reminds us, "Friends come in all shapes and sizes. A true friend really gets you. They like you, flaws and all. They know what to say, and more importantly, when to say nothing at all. When you flip through the collage of people in your life, you may have some people in your corner that you can count on; you may have a band of merry men; you may even have the benefit of a best friend who is there with you to the end. Choose your friends wisely, and that's one of the best ways to level up in life. The opposite is also true.

A Lifetime of People

When I look back on the fifty years of my life and reflect on the many friends who have shared my journey, I recall so many friends who have touched my life in so many ways. When I pause to think about an entire lifetime, I realize the many gifts I have received over the years.

Reflecting back, I realize even the people who challenged me the most helped create the person I am today. At the time I may have been angry with them, but I now realize they were just another kind of angel here to give me new lessons and new gifts – to shape my identity and create a foundation of strength. They were divine tests of my true identity. It is easy to say you are kind, compassionate, loving, and wise when life is easy, but life will send you tests to determine if you really mean it.

Many of us have heard the phrase "people come into our life for a reason, a season, or a lifetime." People can change our lives. Even a chance meeting with a stranger can create a momentary friendship. There is magic in noticing and savoring those moments of friendship whether it's for a brief encounter, an era in time, or an entire life.

Girls' Night Out – *Creating Magic in an Evening*

Christmas seems to come faster each year. Shopping for gifts, setting up the tree, and planning the Christmas vacation week from school all take time. Sometimes I crave a break from the chaos. They say, "It takes a village." Who are "they" anyway? I'd love a village, but I will settle for some time with my girlfriends. I was sure they were doing the same thing for their families! This year I would find some time, even if only for an evening. It was Tuesday and I sent emails and left messages for several of my friends to come over on Thursday. To my surprise, most of them could make it. Many of them did not know each other, and I hoped they would connect and enjoy the evening. We all brought food, drinks, and good holiday cheer. As the evening progressed, it was the typical chatter about the holidays, children, vacation plans, and similar superficial chit-chat. As we sat around the table, I shared my magical moments tradition and asked each person to share a magical moment in their life.

"My two-year-old son had his first Christmas show, and it was joyful to see him onstage. In class, he is so animated and loves to sing and dance, but when the curtain went up for the show, he just stood still there, dazed and dazzled by the crowd! It was adorable. I can't wait for him to see the video when his is older. I realized how quickly my little guy will grow up!"

"Everyone thinks my job is glamorous, and they tell me how lucky I am. Frankly, I don't love my job; it is really challenging and I don't want it anymore. My magical moment was having a break from work to take a walk to the beach. On my way back, the sun broke through the clouds. I stood there for a few moments absorbing the warmth from the beautiful sunlight. That for me is a real magical moment!"

"My oldest son suffers from mental health challenges, and we spend a great deal of time, energy, and resources on his medical care. It drains us emotionally and financially. Yet last week he called to tell me he loves me and is grateful for all that I have done for him. It is rare that he tells me he loves me and even more rare that he shows any gratitude. Those magical moments are special treasures I keep in my heart to carry me through his frequent emotional swings."

"Both of my teenage sons live for hockey. They both live away from home so they can play on nationally ranked teams. My magical moment was flying to a game where they played against each other! I remember when they were little boys playing with their hockey sticks outside. Just sitting in those stands made me realize the value of cherishing the moments each year of our life."

"My father's dementia is getting worse and worse. He barely recognizes anyone anymore. I pray constantly for him. My magical moment was when we visited him recently and for a brief moment he recognized me. God gave me one more moment to tell my dad I love him."

After the last person shared their magical moment, we all seemed to sit in sacred silence cherishing the thoughts, joys, even the sorrows that emerged from this brief get-together. Since that night, this group of mothers has emailed me regularly seeking another night together with that "village" of women.

A Reason

You never know when a moment spent talking to someone can turn into a life-changing event. There is a beautiful quote by an unknown author that says, "Being kind is much more important than being right, for sometimes what a person needs isn't a brilliant mind that speaks but rather a patient heart that listens." These next two stories illustrate this sentiment perfectly.

Take a Moment to Save a Life – Lyn's Story

Today is over and I would like to share how special it has been. I looked into the waiting room and there sat a man with his head in his hands. I asked if he needed an appointment, and he looked up and said, "I was here two weeks ago and you sat and talked with me in the stairwell about life and challenges. What you didn't know was that I was planning to kill myself when I went home. You are an angel with invisible wings."

I don't know how many souls I have saved, and it's not important. What I now know and I truly understand is why things happen for me, not to me. There is magic in our lives every moment of every day – all we have to do is be aware of it and appreciate every moment in this life.

The Power Is On! – Kevin's Story

What started out as a typical day became one of the greatest gifts in my life… a gift that impacted people who were once strangers, as well as my family. I was having lunch at Whole Foods and an elderly couple in their eighties was sitting next to me, just within earshot. The woman was listening and was visibly anxious while her husband spoke on the phone to the gas and electric company about their electric bill, which apparently hadn't been paid for a couple of months. He was explaining to them that they were trying to sell their house, and that's why they couldn't pay their bill. They just didn't have the money. From his response, it was apparent they were telling him he had to pay or they were going to shut him off. His wife began to cry as he hung up the phone.

I felt such compassion for the couple and was compelled to do something to help. I tapped the wife on the shoulder and said, "Ma'am, I couldn't help but overhear about your electrical bill. I think we should do something about it. I'd like to take you to the PG&E office and see if we can't get your bill lowered. I'd like to pay it. I don't think it's right that you have no power and it's causing you such grief. I'd like to help." They were foreign, with an accent, and couldn't believe it.

They followed me to the gas and electric company office where I told the manager, "I'd like to pay their bill, but I'd like to see it adjusted so it is affordable and they can make a reasonable payment every month." The manager hadn't experienced anything like this before and was inspired. He was able to cut their bill in half, which I paid. As they were leaving, I went to them and said, "I just want you to go home and not worry anymore. Turn the lights on. Watch television. Turn the heat on. Just relax. The check here is for next month. Just turn the lights on again, watch TV, and relax. You've lived a long, good life, and it's important not to be stressed." They gave me an email address and a big hug.

I went home, and my wife, Valerie, asked, "Why are you late?" I told her, "I had to go pay someone's electrical bill." And she looked at me and said, "What do you mean, somebody else's electrical bill? You mean our electrical bill?" I said, "No, it was somebody else's. They really needed some help at this time in their lives." Then she looked into my eyes and she got it. She got it right away. The good had been done.

I got in touch with them a couple of weeks later to see how everything was going, and also to ask if they needed another check to help get them through. They said, "We want to have you and your wife and kids over for lunch." My initial reaction was that I didn't want them to spend any money on a lunch for my family, yet we agreed to come.

We went to their house and their "children" were there to meet us. The "kids" were in their sixties and were all there to greet my family and "the person who had helped them through their hard times." They couldn't believe that someone had done that. We told stories during lunch and just talked about our lives. And we became friends. We left five hours later with full bellies and full hearts. I heard from one of the children that sometimes their mom didn't have enough money for gas, so I tried to offer her $20 privately so she could get gas and continue to drive around. But she said, "No, no. I have something for YOU." She gave me an envelope and told me, "Open the card on your way home."

It was a magical afternoon. We took home apples that we picked from their garden and a couple of bottles of wine from their winery, made from grapes they had grown. After giving everybody hugs, we left. On the way home, I opened the envelope, and inside was a beautiful thank-you note about how appreciative they were for our humanity. In it was cash... all the money that we had lent them. And it said, "The house is probably going to sell, and we wanted to give you your money back because we always do that. And that's the right thing to do."

The magic for me was the purity of just giving when someone was really down and directly affecting their lives. I didn't care who saw it or who knew about it. It was just me and them and the moment we shared. I was nervous about it at first. I didn't have the money to give. But there was somebody in greater need than I, and knowing that somebody else was going to have a good month was such a great feeling, so honest and simple. It felt wonderful just doing the right thing.

When we take the time to listen carefully to others, we are able to offer support and friendship in a variety of ways. A good friend is always willing to listen, and a good friend will take the time to show others that they care. Sometimes these acts of kindness can be extended to strangers, and new friendships can be born.

REFLECT

- When was the last time someone in your life paused to listen to you, really listen to you, and show you how much they care about you?
- When was the last time you paused to listen, really listen, and show a friend you really care?

A Season

Traditions with friends and families are one of the key things children remember as they grow up. It's those repetitive things that people do together that create memories of magical moments. They create the unique makeup of friends and families together. If you ask my adult children what they remember about their childhood, they will most likely start with their memories of time with friends and family at our annual family camp.

Annual Camping Trip at the Lair – *Camp Blue Campers*

We drive for hours on the freeway, then exit and drive another few hours, as the towns get smaller and smaller. Next we pass through farmland, and then we begin the ascent up the mountain. The vast dry fields are replaced with beautiful pine trees and views from the valleys and mountain ranges. Then we see the sign reading "Camp Blue Road" and we know we have arrived. Yet another year at our family camp with friends we see but once a year. Week 9 - Tent 55 – our home for a week. Our family of seven fits into a 12x12 tent at the same place and same time every year. We are home.

We've watched our children grow from babies to college students. We have shared much laughter and fun at our evening campfire shows. We've held our breath as we watched our children jump off the cliffs into Pinecrest Lake. We've made pots on the potter's wheels, eaten hundreds of s'mores, hiked every trail around, and played more tournament rounds of ping-pong than we care to remember! We've cheered for the dads at the Big Softball Game on Friday against Camp Gold next door. We've survived cancers, divorces, illnesses, raising children, and even the dreaded teens! We've grieved the campers that have passed on. Sunday Morning Creekside sets the tone for the week where we share our moments from the year, our lessons, our loves, our losses, and our lives. Then it's the Wacky Pool Show, root beer floats, spoon diving for the kids, and inner-tube water polo for the men! Monday is Disco Bingo. Wednesday is the Camper Talent Show. Lots to cheer about. Nothing changes: that's the magic of our family camp. We see mostly the same people each year. We don't know many of their last names, where they live, or what they do for a living. We just know that we are together for this one week in the mountains each year where families live like a village and laugh and spend time outside – magical moments all day – a welcome break from our busy, fast-paced, technologically focused world. No electronics for the kids, just pinecones, open air, and a huge lake. Life is good. Now, how do we bring this magic home?

After twenty-five years at this camp, we know that we will have to wait for these magical moments until the same time next year... and hopefully many more years after that.

REFLECT

- What unique traditions do you share with your friends and family?
- What were some of the magical moments and memories of those times?

- What traditions can you create with your family and friends?

A Lifetime

The words that escape a friend's mouth are "I'll be there when you say you need me," but the words that are unheard from a true friend's heart are "I'll be there...whether you say you need me or not."

Stand By Me – *Greg and Todd's Story*

Lots of people want to ride with you in the limo, but what you want is someone who will take the bus with you when the limo breaks down.

– Oprah Winfrey

The goods times...wine parties, kids born close to one another, sharing the fun of having children, buying the first home, sunsets, days on the beach, memories of the years gone by. Life was good for those years; actually, life was great!

Then things changed. Walking through the aisles of the local Vons, I can still remember the call I made to my good friend.

"Hey."

"Hey, Greg. How are you?"

"I'm getting divorced."

"What?"

"Yeah. Regina told me that she wants to get a divorce."

If I recall correctly, the words came out rather matter-of-factly. At that point the wound had just opened up, fresh. Too soon to really feel the pain that would be forthcoming. Most likely the numbing sensation I felt at the time was due to the shock of finally realizing that I was going to have a failed marriage on my hands.

"Come on over now. Or let's go to Erc's to get a beer. I'm here for you now… and always."

True friendship. At that moment I realized that I had a really great friend. No "I am busy with my own family, or work" or "I don't feel great" excuses; instead, an unequivocal offer of support.

The weeks went by and the misery and pain of divorce came with them. However, the pain was eased by the knowledge that I had my friend Todd – he was, and continues to be, a great ally and a true good friend. He was just there for me. There were many nights that he invited me over to his house for a barbeque, a glass (or two) of wine, a fire in the pit out front, or simply an escape from the hard times that I was going through.

Recently, my mom suddenly found herself in the hospital being rushed in for emergency surgery. I was lucky enough to be with her. When I walked back into the waiting room, there was Todd again, waiting there for me.

A good friend, a really good friend, is special, is magic. When times were really hard he would remind me that things would get better, and in time they did. Yet all through the emotional ups and downs he was there, by my side, in my corner.

I benefitted from his friendship and he asked nothing in return.

Todd took the bus with me when the limo broke down and he continues to be there for me. He defines what it means to be a friend.

A true friend is there for you during the good times and the bad. They will know what to do or say when you are feeling down, or when you need to get out and go on an adventure. It is important to take the time to remember the magical moments we have had with friends throughout the years. By remembering these moments we can experience the immense gratitude that comes with magical friendships. We can contact the people in our lives who have had a big impact and let them know we are thankful for them. We can call them, send them an email or a Facebook message, or even write them a letter.

True friendships are magical, and we should take the time to express our gratitude to those who have blessed us with their love and compassion over the years; in doing so we can create magic in their lives. We can also examine ourselves to see if we have been good friends to others. By being our best selves, we inspire our friends to be the same. And over time some friends become part of the family – part of the indescribably wonderful network that keeps our lives full of magical moments rich with meaning and happiness.

REFLECT

- When was the last time you called a friend, emailed them, sent them a Facebook message or even wrote them a real letter just to let them know how thankful you are for their friendship?
- What would have to happen for you to take a moment today to do that?

Daisy Grows Up – *Suzanne's Story*

> *I feel lucky enough to have magic moments daily from many pieces of my life...when Poppy aged five slips her hand through mine or when my dog puts her head on my shoulder and gives me a dog hug! When light comes through the clouds and it feels like God is saying hello...and many more!*

Nearly twelve years ago my goddaughter, Daisy, was born in Nottingham to great friends of mine, and I saw her several times a week for the first four years of her life; I am privileged to be one of her godparents and have had many beautiful, joyful moments as she progressed from crawling to toddling to walking and beyond.

Daisy would ask her parents if I was coming over and would want to wait up until I arrived and ask me to sleep in her bed or have one last game of whatever it was they were playing with me before she went to sleep.

One day as we were traveling somewhere and I sat in the back of the car with her, she turned to me and said, "I love you, Suze," and then turned away...my heart flipped with love, awe, and gratitude!

When Daisy was four, my company asked me to move away from Newcastle to London, and my boyfriend of some years was also there so I decided to take the opportunity to go (even though it was a wrench to move away from many close friends). When Daisy's mum told her she gave the reason that my boyfriend was in London and I was going to be with him. I have to say I was dreading the conversation with her a little bit as I knew it would be tough moving away from this little sweet loving soul. I had stayed over one night and had slept in the attic room. First thing in the morning she came up to find me (as she often did), and as I got up she stood at the end of the bed and said, "Why do you have to move to London, Suze, I don't want you to go... can your husband not move here?" As you can imagine I was choked as I explained that he couldn't and that I also had to move because of work.

I was in London for three years, and during that time Daisy grew from a toddler to a seven-year-old "teenager" who I loved seeing a few times a year...the bond we had seemed to dwindle during these years as she grew up, and as much as I understood hugely, my heart yearned a little for the bond that once was.

I moved back to Newcastle three years later to live close by to family and be very involved with the horse riding and show jumping that all the girls in the family took part in. I've been blessed to form close bonds with all of them and I love them completely. Daisy had been, and was going through, the journey we all do to establish ourselves outside our family in school and the activities of life. She showed herself to be much more fashion and trend conscious than her sisters and to me was less tactile than the toddler I had played with—she developed a focused character and knew what she wanted. During the journey, and over the next five years, I could be as equally dismissed from the conversation or activity as I could be included (I may be ignored or asked to watch twenty handstands one after the other and judge them...a magic moment, or twenty, in itself!). Either way was appreciated as all part of the journey (Daisy's and mine).

This last year there were a couple of occasions when out of the blue I got my hand held or was given a hug (not usual for the now nearly twelve-year-old Daisy), and they were all magic moments indeed! Then one day out of the blue at the end of a horse show, at which Daisy had much success, she came to me and asked if she could travel home in the car with me, to which of course I said yes! Then she gave me a huge hug and with a great big gorgeous smile said, "Thanks for all your help, Suze, thanks for everything!"

My heart flipped as Daisy gave me a wonderful magic moment, reminding me that bonds are never broken...they are easily renewed. This moment also made me think – what we see in others we see in ourselves.

In this moment with Daisy I realized that over the years through my own challenges, growth, and struggles with finding myself and through the dynamics of life I haven't always been as tactile as I could be; I haven't always shown those I care about how much I care, and I have often been too wrapped up in my own journey to notice where others are on their own. What a magical moment she gave me – a great lesson and a great gift.

Loving Our Four-Legged Friends

If having a soul means being able to feel love and loyalty and gratitude, then animals are better off than a lot of humans.

– James Herriot

Pug, Where Is He? – A Dog Lover's Story

When I was a teenager I spent a lot of my time mopping floors and cleaning up after endless numbers of cats and dogs. I worked hard in a veterinary hospital after school to earn my own spending money because my family had limited financial resources.

I liked animals but had never really felt an attachment to one because my interactions with animals had always been short and sterile.

Then one day a woman came in requesting that we put her dog, a pug, to sleep. She felt he was too sick, and too much to care for. She really couldn't afford any more. Dr. Fischer, the veterinarian, told the woman we would take care of it, and he brought the dog to the back of the hospital. He was not the most beautiful dog with his bulging eyes and completely wrinkly face, but there was something about him that said, "Love me." I remember that moment – it was magical. I asked Dr. Fischer if we could help him and he agreed. I creatively named him "Pug."

Pug lived at the veterinary hospital, and each day I would come to work early, leave work late, and spend time on weekends caring for him, bathing him, and walking him. Little by little, Pug became mine. He was still a bit sick, wobbled when he walked, and just wasn't quite right – but I loved him. I guess I really didn't notice him getting sicker and sicker over time. He was just my Pug.

One day I went to work as usual and walked directly back to Pug's kennel. He wasn't there. I ran up to the front office at the hospital and asked, "Where is Pug?" The office staff looked at each other and then at Dr. Fischer, who came out of the office and wrapped his arm around me and told me Pug was gone. He was too sick. It is amazing how much you can love someone, even an animal, and because of that immense love choose not to see the challenges they may face. I was heart broken.

After some time passed, I realized that my time with Pug is a magical gift that has taught me to love our four-legged friends with as much passion and care as anyone in life. Thank you, Pug, for the gift you gave me.

REFLECT

- Have you ever loved an animal?
- Has there ever been an animal that has changed your life or the life of someone you know?
- How can you show animals love and kindness?

7

The Magic of Time Alone

Perhaps, after all, our best thoughts come when we are alone.
It is good to listen, not to voices but to the wind blowing,
to the brook running cool over polished stones,
to bees drowsy with the weight of pollen.
If we attend to the music of the earth, we reach serenity.
And then, in some unexplained way, we share it with others.

– Gladys Taber

One of the most important relationships in life is the relationship we have with ourselves. In order to create magical moments in our life, we have to know, love, and appreciate ourselves. It is important that we spend quality time alone. By strengthening the bond with ourselves, we can better spend quality time with others.

REFLECT

- When was the last time you spent time with yourself and truly enjoyed the pleasure of your own company?
- How can we expect others to love being with us if we haven't taken the time to appreciate and love being with ourselves?
- What would have to happen for you to schedule some time to get to know yourself?

Let Me Introduce You

An important skill to master in life is to enjoy the pleasure of your own company. People rarely take time to be alone and to appreciate who they are in this world.

Can you remember a time when you met a great new friend and were excited to introduce them to someone else? Think of all the things you liked about that person. What did you say about that person? How did you feel when you were with them? What did you admire most about them? What did you enjoy most about spending time with them?

Now, imagine that person is you. What if you felt all those things about yourself? Imagine feeling such admiration and respect for yourself that you were proud to introduce yourself to other people. What would you say about yourself? Do you really know yourself enough to answer that question?

Oftentimes we seek love and respect from others. Remember no one will love and respect you more than you love and respect yourself. The first love affair you must have is a love affair with yourself.

A Sure Thing – *A Date with Yourself*

Years ago when I was single, after many first dates I became weary of the dating life. One evening I called several friends to go out to dinner or meet for a glass of wine downtown. No one was available. After puttering around my house, I decided to go out to dinner on my own. I paused, started to get ready, and thought, "Can I really make a reservation for one?"

I called my favorite San Diego restaurant and did just that. As I dressed, I jokingly said, "I have a date with myself. I am a sure thing and I will be right on time."

A smile crossed my face as I drove to dinner. When I arrived, I announced to the maître d' that I was taking myself on a date and would he please seat me at a wonderful table with a kind and attentive waiter. After a laugh and a kindhearted smile, he ushered me to the table and directed the wait staff to take exceptional care of me – which indeed they did.

I had a memorable and lovely meal. I felt well cared for and thoroughly enjoyed the pleasure of my own company. This began my tradition of dates with myself.

It has been years since that first date. I am happily married to the man of my dreams, have five wonderful and loving children, and a dog named Buddy. Yet I maintain that tradition, and on many nights a year you will find me happily creating magical moments and enjoying the pleasure and magic of time with myself.

REFLECT

- What ways can you enjoy the pleasure of your own company? Here are a few ideas (be sure to come up with some of your own):
    - Create a special place for you to spend time with yourself at home.
    - Take yourself on a lunch or dinner date.
    - Plan an entire day of things you love to do.
    - Write a letter to someone telling them about this great person in your life: you!
    - Make a list of things you can do to appreciate yourself and then do one a week.
    - Write in a journal all the reasons you are grateful for who you are in this life.
    - Write your life story – it is only partway done; compose the second half and make yourself the hero.

Carefree Playful Fun

If people never did silly things,
nothing intelligent would ever get done.

– Ludwig Wittgenstein

When was the last time you did something carefree, playful, and fun on your own? Take the time to enjoy your own company and you will find that you can have immense fun by yourself.

Real Men Watch Kids' Movies – *Scott's Story*

I am a professional man and entrepreneur. I am a football and basketball referee. Some people refer to me as a "jock." I golf with friends and enjoy a superb glass of red wine on occasion.

Much of my day is spent focusing on my career and expanding my business. I am an avid sports fan and can easily immerse myself in a day of NFL football games with friends.

Yet one afternoon I enjoyed a different outing. I drove myself to the local movie theater, bought buttered popcorn and a soda, and settled in to watch the latest kids' film, The Lego Movie. I laughed hysterically, experienced pure carefree fun, and thoroughly enjoyed this outing with myself. The laughter from the kids in the audience carried me away to a faraway time when life was simpler and playful times were easy.

I look forward to The Lego Movie sequel for my next magical moment on my own!

REFLECT

- When was the last time you experienced playful carefree fun?
- What activities can you do that will make you feel this way?
- What would have to happen for you to schedule this "fun" each week?

Do What You Love and Friends Will Come

In the well-known book *Do What You Love and the Money Will Follow*, author Marsha Sinetar explains how to follow your heart to make a living. The same principle applies here. Do what you love doing and the right friends and people will come into your life to support you.

The Secret Spot in Ireland – Nick's Story

My magical moment happened the first day of my solo surf trip to Ireland. Each year I go to different spots around the world to surf. I often go by myself, and in those moments alone I have been fortunate enough to have new friends appear in my life.

On this particular day, I woke up early and set out to go surfing. I had no real map or directions but I knew where the ocean was, so I just started driving in that direction. After driving by myself on highways, side roads, dirt roads, trails, and through farmland, I eventually ended up at the ocean and what appeared to be the perfect surf spot. There was no one else around for miles in any direction.

After thirty minutes of debating whether or not I should go out by myself, I was about to leave when a car with four other Irish surfers pulled up. We started chatting and they told me that somehow I had managed to discover a secret awesome surf spot that very few people knew about. They said they were going to paddle out and asked me if I wanted to join them. Having traveled thousands of miles just to get there, I jumped at the chance.

After surfing for a while and catching some amazing waves, I sat there for a moment and thought to myself how magical and amazing it was that I was thousands of miles from home, sitting in the ocean in the middle of nowhere, and surfing a spot that almost no one knew about with my new friends. After surfing for several hours we all came in and the Irish guys invited me to join them at the local pub where we drank Guinness and swapped surf stories. A secret surf spot, new Irish friends, and Guinness made for some truly magical moments.

REFLECT

- What do you love to do?
- What would have to happen for you to enjoy doing these things on your own?

- What would have to happen for you to pursue these experiences now?
- What if you trusted that the right people will come to support you when the time is right?

Gratitude for Your Body, Mind, and Spirit

Your body, mind, and spirit are with you your whole life. They are always your most faithful servants, even when you don't always care for them or treat them well.

When was the last time you spent some time with yourself, really getting to know who you are and how best to take care of your true self? You will be amazed at the messages your body, mind, and spirit give you, leading you to a healthier and happier life.

All I Need Is in Me Now – *A Meditator's Story*

We often seek fulfillment and happiness outside of ourselves. We often want the next best thing, and too often when we get it we immediately focus on the next thing. Many of us get onto that treadmill of life and don't know how to get off it. I know, because I ran that treadmill and became exhausted from stress, pressure, and life's challenges: career, family, and finances.

At one point I just needed a break. Lucky for me, at the right time I was given a gift. I was able to attend Deepak Chopra's signature event "Seduction of Spirit" at the Chopra Center. I went to escape the day-to-day stress of my life, and I really had no clue what the event would be about. When I arrived, I realized this event was a five-day immersion into meditation.

I said to myself, "This should be interesting. I can barely sit still, let alone quiet the thoughts in my mind." I knew no one at the event and really wanted time to be alone and escape my life. Each day we would gently meditate several times, and as the days progressed I felt my body relaxing and my mind quieting ever so slightly.

On the last day, after one of the meditations, I felt my body saying, "Please don't stop; this finally feels right."

So began my love affair with the quiet, peace, and solitude that meditation brings into my life. I learned the important skill of paying attention to my body and the inner voice that becomes buried due to our modern, technologically advanced, fast-paced lives. There are days my body is tired, so I welcome the sleep during meditation. There are days when I appreciate the gift of just noticing my thoughts (good or challenging) as they come and go during meditation. There are days that I merely focus on my rhythmic breathing or mantras as I relax into a safe and quiet place. There are also days when I am carried away into the sacred space where there is no time and no space – the gap between my thoughts.

I learned from that event that all the peace and well-being I really need is in me always. Sometimes you just need to pause and learn to be with the silence. Years later as my meditation practice has progressed, I still feel that same feeling. Some days I feel turbulence inside. Some days I am restless. Some days I am tired. Most of all, I have learned that my body will tell me what it needs if I just pause to listen. I have been blessed to become a meditation instructor for the Chopra Center and share this wonderful gift with others. I know that I can always find magical moments if I take the time to meditate.

REFLECT

- How do you nurture and care for your body, mind, and spirit.
- What could you do to treat yourself even better?

- Do you appreciate the messages your body gives you?
- Your body constantly communicates with you. Gut feelings start the dialogue with your inner voice. Do you listen to that dialogue and act accordingly?
- Can you remember the last time your heart and spirit told you to do one thing, yet you did another?

Who Are You?

In order to experience magic, you should know yourself. We all should take the time to be alone and discover who we truly are. We need to be aware of what we tell ourselves so that we can master our emotions and live and love in good health in mind, body, and spirit.

Outrageous Soul – *A Man's Declaration*

Some people say I am outrageous. I like it that way. I have earned the right to be anything I want. I have been on the brink of bankruptcy and worked my way back to success with the help of a lot of awesome people in my life. I live a life of extreme gratitude, and I only hope to inspire others to do the same. I give back to my employees, my community, and others in the work I do serving people in the personal development world.

I live my own life and if you want to come along – awesome. Be ready for fun and be ready for anything. There are people who watch life happen, there are people who make life happen, and there are people who wonder what happened. Come along on my ride if you are ready to MAKE your life happen.

As the international peak performance coach Anthony Robbins has said, "The words you say with emotional intensity become your life—it can be your heaven or your hell." I choose heaven, although on occasion I do like to stir up some hell.

I want to be known as a man who walks his talk. But before I can walk it, I have to know my talk. And I have to mean it. This certainly doesn't mean walking someone else's talk or listening to the banter of other people's ideas of who I am or what I should do. I am in control of my own life.

I live my magic each day in each moment with every breath I take. If I were to name one magical moment a day, it would be my daily incantation. I can say it in my sleep as I live it with my every breath. I say it with passion when I work out and when I drive my car. It is ingrained in me and it lifts me up when I am challenged.

Here is my outrageous soul and my daily incantation bare on this paper for all of you to read. Hopefully you will be inspired to write your own:

> *I, Woody, see, hear, feel, and know that the purpose of my life is to be a passionate, loving, outrageous soul who empowers myself and others to be their very best. I believe in expanding possibilities and living my dreams no matter what. With my faith, my determination, and my self-confidence I can overcome and defy any odds. Let the abundance of our universe flow freely through my veins. I am one with God and God is one with me. Yes, I am gifted. Yes, I am guided. Yes, I am certain because I decided. Today I will be grateful, thankful, and unstoppable!*

REFLECT

- What words do you say to yourself and others with emotional intensity on a regular basis?
- Do you have a daily incantation?
- Are there words you tell yourself that help you live the best version of yourself?

- How do these mantras help you know yourself?
- Take the time to write a daily incantation that reaffirms the positive aspects of your personality. Say this to yourself with emotional intensity and conviction every day. Feel it in your body and radiate it through your spirit to continually remind yourself of how awesome you are.

These next two stories illustrate the power of learning and knowing who we are.

A Fork in the Road – *A Teen's Decision*

> *I think that somehow, we learn who we really are*
> *and then live with that decision.*
>
> *– Eleanor Roosevelt*

A sunny afternoon, trade winds blowing, a shimmering sun dances on the tropical water. Diamond Head looms behind me, somehow watching the waves and surfers who ride the swell, day after day, year after year. The boards change with the outfits people wear to the beach, but this beautiful outcropping of hardened magma stares and keeps watch.

Bobbing up and down in the ocean, waiting for the next wave to hit the reef, break, and allow me to ride it, I sit and reflect on thirty years of surfing. Has it been that long since I first borrowed a purple and green pin-tailed board that belonged to a friend and attempted to paddle into the ocean? Thirty years of riding waves, living and breathing as a surfer, identifying myself as a surfer, being inspired by watching the ocean and the waves that reach the shores wherever I happen to be. It almost seems impossible to imagine a life that didn't involve surfing. When do we decide who we will become? Is this a cognitive decision that a fourteen-year-old is even capable of making?

As with most American youth, I too grew up playing the sports that we are accustomed to playing. Fall meant joining another AYSO soccer team. Winter meant youth basketball, and spring, well, of course meant baseball. I started my athletic career when I was six. By the time I was ten, I was playing soccer and baseball. By thirteen, soccer, basketball, and baseball. Summer was beach time. Volleyball, boogie boarding, bodysurfing, lying around with pals at Fourth, Fifth, and later Seventh streets. My dad was a great athlete having had success in baseball and football. My brother was a very good baseball and soccer player. Thus the expectation in my family was that I too would follow in these footsteps and continue the proud tradition of American youth playing "American" sports. All the while my destiny would throw a fork in the road. A choice.

August 1984. I had begun my high school career. Summer ended early when I had to go to Mira Costa High School and begin "two-a-days." Dreaded by football players the world over, two-a-days refers to double practices with tons of running in the midst of August, perhaps the hottest time of the year. I decided to play football because I was born with broad shoulders, was strong, and was fairly athletic. Football, as seen as a path, stretched along the road of American sports. I had been on this path for eight years by the time football began. I played football because I was expected to play football, soccer, and, in the spring, baseball. I was following the path that American boys are expected to follow, a trail well worn in the fabric of American history. (I should probably say here that recent history has seen a dramatic shift away from the three-sport athlete. Today, high school athletes specialize in one sport. They play for the high school in season, then on club teams for the rest of the year.) The football experience was an interesting one for me. It took me totally out of my comfort zone. I was hit and had to hit back. I had to learn plays that made no sense to me. I had to run, jump, tackle, and get yelled at by coaches (who should have been called "yellers" for the utter lack of teaching that went on). Needless to say, on many days I would see my friends heading off to the beach while I was heading off to a place my fourteen-year-old brain could see only as a place of pain.

I think my subconscious pointed me toward my path early on in my football career. Toward the end of two-a-days, I missed practice and went surfing at a famous surf spot called San Onofre. My friends Bryan and Eric also played football and also thought the experience was horrific. We ditched football and went surfing. We paid a terrible price for those six hours of surfing pleasure, but I look back now and realize that my body and mind were showing me the way toward my future.

Mercifully, football ended in early November. Having won a game, yes one game, I was thankful that I could now look forward to some free time after school. Winter was an enjoyable time of surfing, school, and hanging out with friends. Winter in Manhattan Beach means cold water, but it is also a time when the large Pacific storms create the swells that move the sand around and create better waves. However, expectations were that I would try out for baseball and continue along the chosen path...the path of traditional American sports. My dad had talked to the baseball coach and was informed that I would have to try out, but there would likely be a place for me on the team.

Monday came. Sixth period. Tryouts. I can still remember walking down the ramp. Cleats on. Mitt in hand. Backpack on.

Little did I know that on that day I had come to a fork in the road. Little did I know that I was about to make a decision that not only defined who I was, but also who I became. Another view might be that on that day, in February 1984, I simply made a snap decision and only later realized that I had decided who I was and who I wanted to become. Regardless of how I see it now, on that day I saw a good friend who told me that the waves were going off (meaning "the waves are really good"). I looked at the baseball field and looked down the ramp. Ramp meant surfing. Baseball field meant, well, baseball. I can remember thinking that my dad would be mad that I was blowing off baseball to surf. If I missed tryouts, I was not playing baseball.

I can remember to this day, twenty-nine years later, that I simply put my mitt back into my backpack and walked on down the ramp toward home, toward surfing. It would be nice to say that my step was a little lighter, my face brightened by the knowledge that I had pursued a path I wanted to pursue; but I don't know if in fact that was true. Probably the reality was that my step was heavier knowing that I had decided to do something that went against family expectations, and that I would have to explain to my dad that I didn't go to baseball and chose to surf instead.

What I do know looking back is that I made a decision that came from my soul. It was a decision that changed my life and helped to define me as an individual. When I look back to that day in February 1984, that decision stands as a significant fork in the road of life.

You sow a habit and reap a character. You sow a character and reap a destiny. Anon.

So true.

My Victory: Sunrise at Donner Lake – *A Triathlete's Story*

When I was in sixth grade, my friends and I decided it would be really fun to try out for the junior high school girls' softball team together. We went and bought mitts and cleats. We showed up for tryouts all ready to play on the team and have a fun season being together. After many cuts had been made, on the last day of tryouts, the coaches were making the final team decision – only two more cuts. At the end of the day, we were all excited to look at the final team roster. After school, I rushed to look at the board outside the locker room. I wasn't on the list. I couldn't believe the coach cut me from the team. Devastation… When I went to talk to Coach Hansen, she told me I didn't open my mitt enough to catch balls and I couldn't hit. I was stunned!

In that moment, at eleven years old, I decided I was not an athlete.

Over the next few years in junior high school, friends would invite me to play soccer, swim, or play volleyball and other sports. I would make excuses and decline their offers…I wasn't an athlete.

Then high school – opportunities for sports came and went again. I took a pass on all of them; I WASN'T AN ATHLETE.

As an adult, I would work out in the gym – not everyone in the gym was an athlete. Running on the treadmill, riding the stationary bike, and occasionally lifting some weights – those were just good health decisions.

After my third child was born, my body needed to recover. Over that prior three-year period, I had two very challenging pregnancies that required some intense medical attention. The specialists decided that I needed to be on bed rest for my pregnancies. "You mean I really have to stay lying down for all that time?"

After my daughter Samantha was born, my body was tired and worn out. I did not have a lot of stamina or strength. I needed to regain my energy back. At first I could barely walk to the end of our block without someone slowly helping me along. After some time, I could walk a bit farther but it was really a strain.

After a couple of months of every day moving a little more and more, I was able to start going to the gym again. I could actually move my body again. Short walks on the treadmill became short runs and then longer. Fifteen minutes on the stationary bike turned into thirty then an hour... maybe a spin class here and there.

Then one night, my new friend Katie invited us over for dinner. When we arrived, the first thing I noticed was the bike leaning against the table in her living room. It was a high-tech road bike – amazing, thin, light as a feather. When I asked her about it, Katie shared her stories and passion about being a triathlete. I sat there listening in awe – WOW – my friend was a real triathlete... that was something incredible! I was mesmerized hearing about her adventures and stories about her triathlete friends, her triathlon team, and the experiences at her races: swimming in open water, lakes and oceans... biking and running on mountain ranges, coastline, and in amazing towns and cities.

At that dinner, I shared how challenging it was getting my strength back after my pregnancies, how I slowly worked my way back to the gym – struggling to find energy, some days with NO motivation.

Katie then said the magic words, "Why don't you train for a triathlon?"

I instantly responded, "Oh, I am not an athlete..."

Thinking back now, it was interesting how the words just spilled out of my mouth without even thinking about what I was saying.

Katie pressed on. "What do you mean? You run and bike already at the gym – just get in the water and swim...no big deal."

Without hesitation, I said, "It's not who I am. I'm not an athlete and surely not a triathlete – I just go to the gym to stay in good health. I could never compete in a race."
"Why not?" she said.

I didn't have an answer… I couldn't really say, "because I didn't open my mitt when I was eleven and I can't hit a softball." No, I didn't have an answer… I let that question simmer for the next few days.

Why did I automatically say no?

What was the big deal?

One morning, I casually searched for some triathlons just to see what it was all about. I noticed that a local community center was sponsoring a very short sprint distance triathlon.

¼ mile swim in a pool. Could I swim laps?
11-mile bike ride – how long was that on a stationary bike?
5k run – 3.1 miles – I ran longer on the treadmill.

Three months away… I think I could do that … hmmm…

One thing at a time…

First, focus on swimming again – just get in the pool and start, one lap at a time…

Get off the stationary bike and onto a real bike – I could do that. I learned as a kid. What's that phrase? "It's like riding a bike, you always know how…"

Run – what's the real difference between a treadmill and outside? Just do it. I could be the Nike commercial. Okay, here it goes... one step at a time... one block at a time...one mile at a time...

Then... one race at a time...

Community Center Sprint Triathlon... Check!
San Jose International Triathlon... Check!
UVAS Triathlon... Check!
Then another, then another, then another... Check! Check! Check!

I was a triathlete...

Then some friends told me about the triathlon at Donner Lake, a 1.5k swim at 6000 feet elevation in 64-degree water temp, a 40k bike ride up to a 7200-foot elevation at the summit—you climb up narrow switchbacks to the summit, down the backside, and then back up to the summit again, and a 10k run all the way around the lake...hmmm. They told me it was a really challenging race.

Well, back to training...more swimming, this time training in even more open water, one stroke at a time, more biking...this time in altitude and mountains, one pedal stroke at time...then running... endless running...in the mountains...anywhere and anytime I could find time...one step after another. Just do it ...Nike should pay me for my thoughts...

Then race morning came. I had all my gear together...my number was marked on my arms and legs with a big black Sharpie. My children had their posters made reading "Go Mom Go." I drove in the dark early morning hours to Donner Lake, set up in the transition area...wetsuit, goggles on...bike and running gear all laid out and waiting. The other triathletes were warming up and setting up. Excitement was in the air...music, energy, and anticipation swirling around and landing on me and everyone else!

Finally, the loudspeaker announced my heat…time to get in the 64-degree water! The cold water is always a good wakeup call. Swim a few strokes to warm up the body.

I'm ready…I'm floating, I'm waiting…and then I watched the most amazing light as the sun rose over the Donner Pass Mountains. The shining light slowly moved over the swimmers, and you could hear a gasp from everyone in the water. As I floated in the water feeling the sunshine on me, I suddenly realized "I AM AN ATHLETE! I AM REALLY AN ATHLETE! I WAS WRONG ALL THOSE YEARS! I AM REALLY AND TRULY AN ATHLETE! I DON'T NEED A MITT OR A BASEBALL BAT OR A COACH TO TELL ME WHO I AM…I DECIDE WHO I AM! Swim one arm into the water after the other, bike one pedal stroke after another, run one step at a time…go, go, go… I AM AN ATHLETE!"

I was in such bliss that I almost missed the sound of the horn and the start of the race!

Fully embodied in my athlete identity, I dove in Donner Lake embraced by the beautiful light of the sunrise and my shining moment. The fresh water washed my joyful tears away. I pedaled up Donner Pass as if some divine force lifted me and carried me up the mountain. A lighter, brighter step carried me on my run around the lake. As I neared the last turn, the athletes that already finished the race were cheering me on as they had done many races before, but this time it really meant something special. As I crossed through the finish line I dove into the water washing away any belief that would not remind me that I WAS AN ATHLETE. That day was victory…

Embracing Change

Sometimes change in life can at first seem challenging. When faced with life changes, many of us look for what is wrong and what will be missing in our life after the change. Sometimes embracing that change and focusing on what could be possible can lead to life-changing magical moments and even lead to defining who we are in this world.

Time for a Change – *Embracing New Opportunities*

It happened again, suddenly without any warning. My whole life was going to change again. I would leave what I had known for the past seven years to start a new life, meet new people, and go to a new school. Throughout my life I have had to move to different places. It is very hard on me. I can be a very shy person when I meet new people. I have moved from San Francisco to San Diego to Manhattan Beach, California, in my lifetime. I remember being seven years old and my mom saying to me, "We are moving to San Diego." I remember the feeling of being crushed in sadness, like my whole life just suddenly changed for the worse. I did not want to move. I would have to leave my friends and go to a place where I had no connections. It happened again when I was thirteen years old and I moved to Manhattan Beach. I was scared to go to a new high school where I knew no one.

With each new move, I learned that my life could change for the better. Through my fear, I never could have imagined that moving to a new place could give me so many opportunities in life. My magical moments are knowing that I have met people I will have friendships with my whole life, new opportunities that have helped my basketball career drastically, and an entirely new view of life. I have learned that change can be a good thing and it can give you better opportunities in life if you are open to change and make the best use of those opportunities.

When I first moved to San Diego I was nervous because I knew nobody and had never been to Southern California. I was seven years old and it was the first day of school in a new city. I was terrified. I stepped in the classroom knowing nobody. It felt horrible. I felt like I was an outcast in an unknown place. At seven, I was not sure that anyone would be friendly. Thankfully, I met people and started to create new friendships. Miss Taylor, my third-grade teacher, was one of those special people who truly took the time to care for each of her students. She helped introduce me to other kids in the class and gave me the gift of place in that new school.

When I was ten, I probably had the most important encounter of my life. I met Alex Caceres, my basketball coach. He introduced me to the game and I never looked back. Alex grew up in Queens, New York, and grew up playing basketball with many now famous NBA basketball stars. He played serious street ball on some of the most famous courts in New York. He became my mentor in basketball and would change my life forever. With his mentoring and guidance from that point on, basketball was my passion. Alex lives and breathes basketball. He plays with leadership, intensity, passion, and a serious commitment for winning. Alex taught me to play hard and play smart. When I moved again to Manhattan Beach, California, Alex drove there regularly and helped me earn my place in many of the adult pickup games on the courts in Los Angeles. We played together and Alex taught me the ropes in earning my place playing serious street ball. In some of the games on the outskirts of town, I was nicknamed "O."

As time passed in my new home, the same thing happened. I met new people and new coaches that would give me new opportunities in my life. Now I have the chance to play college basketball. It has always been my dream, and it is starting to become a reality—a true magical moment. Looking back, at age seven I was convinced change and moving were bad things. Through my expe-

riences I learned that change can be good, and embracing that belief can change your life for the better. Change can give you the opportunities in life that can help you succeed and even become a better person. It certainly did for me.

Spending time on our own and getting to know ourselves is one of the best things we can do to create magic in our lives. We have to know the power and beauty within ourselves if we are going to be able to share it with other people. We need to explore our inner selves and learn to listen to our inner dialogues. This is one of the greatest gifts we can give to the world. As Sir Thomas Browne says, "All wonders you seek are within yourself." Let's take the time to discover our own treasures.

8

The Magical Gifts in Nature

I love to think of nature as an unlimited broadcasting station through which God speaks to us every hour, if we will only tune in.

– George Washington Carver

Experiencing Our Environment

Adi Shankara, a beloved eighth-century Vedic sage, taught that our physical body includes not just our individual self but also encompasses our environment. Shankara explained that we are in constant interchange with our environment and the world we live in through the air we breathe, the food we eat, the water we drink, and even those around us. Through that continual exchange we become part and parcel of our environment and the world we live in. Shankara reminds us to respect and honor that part of us that we call our physical world.

There is a primal part of us that draws us to nature. We are intimately connected to nature, and nature's rhythms flow within us. Notice how our sleep patterns follow the rising and setting of the sun. Notice how the inflow and outflow of our breath follows the gentle dialogue between the ocean's surf and sand. It is no real wonder that we are drawn to nature, especially in times of stress. Like a lullaby, we just appreciate and experience nature's sounds for the vibrational soothing quality they have on us. Nature is ever changing and flowing; there is a magical quality in nature that takes us back to our primal roots.

There is so much magic in nature. We can experience that magic any time we choose just by pausing to notice it all around us.

Jewels…Bahamas Passage – Randy's Story

> When I was on active duty with the navy, the submarine I was stationed aboard went through a yearlong overhaul. Once we were free of the shipyard, we sailed to the Bahamas for post-overhaul testing. Weapons testing took place on the Atlantic side of the Bahamas and SONAR testing took place on the US side. The transit from one side to the other was too shallow to make submerged. We had to go on the surface.

Modern submarines were made to travel submerged, not on the surface. When they're on the surface, the officer of the deck must be at the top of the "sail" at all times. The sail is that tall part of the submarine that sticks out of the water when the vessel is surfaced. A large, watertight hatch takes up virtually all the standing room, and when the hatch is open, there really isn't any place to sit. The edge of the hatch, while wide, has too many gears and moving parts to be comfortable as a seat. And there is only a three- to four-inch-wide ledge around the hatch opening – not enough to actually stand on. All in all, it's a pretty miserable experience.

Luck was not with me on this particular voyage – or so I thought. I drew the short straw and was on watch as officer of the deck for the entire surface transits from one side of the Bahamas to the other. To make matters worse, they were all made between midnight and 6 a.m. to save daylight hours for running the various tests we were conducting.

So, on the first transit, there I was at the top of the sail. It was pitch black. It was uncomfortable. There was no place to stand. There was nothing to do but stare into the blackness and wait for six interminable hours to pass.

After a while, my eyes adjusted and I began to make out a horizon. The sea was a slightly darker shade of black than the sky. Then I realized the sky wasn't black at all; there were more stars in the heavens than I ever knew existed. It was like God had taken handfuls of luminescent sand and thrown them across the sky over and over and over again. Every star was separate and brilliant.

At some point I looked down at the sea to watch the wake caused by the sail passing through the water. In that part of the world sea algae is phosphorescent—it glows green. The white froth of the water was sprinkled with thousands of "emeralds." As I stared mesmerized into the sea of emeralds, I realized that we were not alone in the ocean. A pod of dolphins had joined us. They were swimming alongside and then began to crisscross in front of us. They stayed for hours.

I was overwhelmed. Every star in creation was over my head. Thousands of "emeralds" were at my feet. And some of the most amazing creatures on the planet were my travel companions. I felt so insignificant in the face of such miraculous creations; so small, so unworthy. And then I realized I was part of all of it.

I didn't tell anyone about my experience. For the next several days I just trudged up to the top of the sail at midnight, where it was dark and uncomfortable, where there was no place to stand, where there was nothing to do, and where there was "nothing" to see. Those nights are some of my most vivid memories, and some of the most magical moments in my life.

The Soul of Water

There is a great healing power in water. About 71 percent of the earth's surface is water. The human body is primarily water. Babies are approximately 78 percent water and the adult body is about 60 percent water. It is no wonder that we are drawn to water. It is a great part of who we are, nourishing us, soothing us, and keeping us alive. The sound of water can heal us. The sight of water calms us. The touch of water can enliven us.

Many of us are drawn to bodies of water for the sight, sound, and feel of water. Water has a power and soul that connects us to this earth. We are water, and this magical and powerful gift of nature continues to provide us with life.

My Lifelong Magical Moment – *A Surfer's Story*

What does surfing mean to me?

Life, expression, connection, soul, style, solitude, excitement, adrenaline, travel, frustration, beauty, waiting, patience, perfection. Someone once said that surfing is like making love. It always feels good no matter how many times you've done it.

Surfing is much more than this; it is an individually unique experience, a sensation, a feeling like hot or cold, pleasure or pain. Surfing, and the experience of being in the ocean, flowing up and down rhythmically, faster or slower, becomes part of your soul.

No one surfing style is exactly the same, as if each of us has a visible fingerprint left on the ocean.

I could tell a thousand magical moment stories that relate to this, but all of these stories are an attempt to put into words the way I feel while immersed in Mother Nature, feeling the natural energy of our world. Could you explain love to someone who has not felt it?

Go surfing...put yourself in the magic of the sea. Experience your own magical moment and you will be in love. Captured like the sailors who hear the siren's song, the moth caught in the glow of the light, the feather caught in the fleeting wind...

Go surfing and leave your magical fingerprint on the sea – then you will create your own magical moments...

The Healing Power of the Mountains

In an article from *Smoky Mountain Living*, the author explains, "The healing power of the mountains has been part of the human psyche for centuries – not just for the psychological benefits, but for actual physical improvements. A prolonged mountain vacation was the standard prescription from doctors in the 1800s and early 1900s for their wealthy patients afflicted with everything from tuberculosis to depression."

Like many people, I am also drawn to the power, serenity, and authenticity of the mountains. Traveling to the mountains brings us closer to the earth, to a deeper reality, a tranquility and peace that you can just feel has been there before our time on this earth. The mountains are something truly real that you can touch, feel, smell, and see beyond the technological life that swirls around us every day at alarming rates.

The Quiet Is Magic – *The Enchanted Dreams Ranch*

I have traveled the world. I have stayed in exceptionally beautiful hotels in more countries than I can count. I have hiked on glaciers in Alaska, safaried in Africa, walked the ancient ruins at Ephesus, floated in the Dead Sea, surfed in Australia, trained with elephants in Thailand, cycled on the back roads of Spain, and so much more.

I found myself thinking about these experiences as I glided back and forth on a simple redwood swing on the front porch of our cabin in the mountains. I was alone enjoying the magic of my memories. As I swung back and forth, I noticed the lovely clouds, the immensity of nature, and the extraordinary quiet all around me.

I had always dreamed of having a place to retreat in my life. In fact, years ago at a county fair, I purchased a wooden sign where I had the artist engrave "Enchanted Dreams Ranch." Over the years as I traveled from place to place, I would imagine if this place or that would someday be my retreat.

Yet one day, as I enjoyed the rocking back and forth on that swing, I realized all the magic I was looking for around the world was right there on that swing on the wooden porch at our cabin in the mountains. My magical moment was realizing it was here all along. As I turned around to see my wooden "Enchanted Dreams Ranch" sign hanging by our front door, I realized it took a lifetime of travel around the world to recognize the magic in a place called home.

Fresh Air, Majestic Mountains, Clear Water –
The Magic of Our Environment

I sit by the side of this lake as I have done time and time again. Yet each time I am still in awe of the smell of the fresh air, the majesty and grandeur in these mountains, the soft breeze on my face, the warm sunshine on my body, and the refreshing feel of clear crisp glistening lake water on my feet. It's such a magical feeling.

It lifts my spirit, fills my soul, and calms my mind, such a welcome respite from the hustle-bustle of the city, the buildings, the cars, the streets, and the day-to-day life that pulls me in so many directions. There are times I forget to pause and take a deep breath in or even to look up at the sky; but at the lake I can slow down and take in all the beauty.

There are so many enriching places in this world, so many places to feel healthy, feel vibrant, and feel alive. Mother Nature has created wonders for us. I am grateful for these moments that connect me even more to the energy and life our world has to offer, if we only just pause to see, hear, and feel its wonder.

REFLECT

- When was the last time you enjoyed yourself in nature?
- When was the last time you breathed in fresh ocean air? Watched a sunset? Listened to the rain? Felt the wind on your body?
- When was the last time you took a moment to appreciate and experience the magic and majesty of the world that surrounds you and is part of you?

Spend time in nature today or this week. It can be as simple as going outside and taking five deep breaths or it can be a journey to sit by the ocean for a few moments matching the flow of your breath to the flow of the water. Watch a sunrise. Look at the moon. Notice the movement of the clouds. Gaze at the stars and take in their beauty. Take the time to discover yourself in nature.

9

Magical Legacies

*Your story is the greatest legacy that you will leave to your friends.
It's the longest-lasting legacy you will leave to your heirs.*

– Steve Saint

The Merriam-Webster dictionary defines legacy as "something… received from an ancestor or predecessor or from the past." Meaningful legacies can be so much more; they can represent the story of someone's life and determine how they are remembered. They can serve as reminders of the lessons they shared and the contributions they made to this world while they were alive.

Sometimes a legacy is represented not only by an experience of how someone lived, but also by how someone died. We read every day about unexpected or tragic deaths. Often the last moments or hours in people's lives leave profound lifelong impressions on all who knew them and even those who didn't.

Unexpected Last Times

Life is what happens when we plan for something else…

9/11 – Legacies for a Nation

For many 9/11 victims, both those that passed away and those that survived, their last moments with their loved ones were on the morning of September 11, 2001. Their daily kisses goodbye, their breakfasts together, and their unresolved issues were all swept away in those tragic moments. They all had unexpected last times.

Life preempts plans. It provides so many unexpected twists and turns that it reminds us to cherish and honor what we have now in the moment.

An unknown author wrote this poem after the tragedy of 9/11.

Last Times

If I knew it would be the last time
that I'd see you fall asleep,
I would tuck you in more tightly
and pray the Lord, your soul to keep.

If I knew it would be the last time
that I'd see you walk out the door,
I would give you a hug and kiss
and call you back for one more.

If I knew it would be the last time
I'd hear your voice lifted up in praise,
I would videotape each action and word,
so I could play them back day after day.

If I knew it would be the last time with you,
I could spare an extra minute or two to stop and say,
"I love you," instead of assuming you would KNOW I do.

If I knew it would be the last time
I would be there to share your day,
Thinking I'm sure you'll have so many more,
so I can let just this one slip away.

For surely there's always tomorrow to make up for an
oversight, and we always get a second chance
to make everything right.

There will always be another day to say our "I love yous,"
and certainly there's another chance to say our
"Anything I can do's?"

But just in case I might be wrong,
and today is all I get,
I'd like to say how much I love you and I hope
we never forget.

Tomorrow is not promised to anyone,
young or old alike,
And today may be the last chance you get
to hold your loved one tight.

So if you're waiting for tomorrow,
why not do it today?
For if tomorrow never comes,
you'll surely regret the day

that you didn't take that extra time
for a smile, a hug, or a kiss
and you were too busy to grant someone,
what turned out to be their one last wish.

So hold your loved ones close today, whisper in their ear.
Tell them how much you love them
and that you'll always hold them dear.

Take time to say, "I'm sorry," "Please forgive me,"
"Thank you" or "it's okay."

And if tomorrow never comes,
you'll have no regrets about today.

– Author Unknown

Many of us remember where we were on 9/11; as we watched the
events unfold, our hearts and prayers went out to the victims and
their families.

I was at a hotel in San Francisco attending a conference when I turned on the television and quickly packed to drive home to my children. I will never forget driving past San Francisco International Airport watching a line of airplanes in the sky preparing to land quickly as our national airspace was immediately cleared.

As my children grew, I cherished the milestones in each of their lives and was grateful each year as they reached adulthood. Watching those planes land, I remembered that the week before, my oldest son, Justin, was having lunch at the World Trade Center with his mentor and close friend David. As I realized he could easily have been in that building on 9/11, I paused and his entire life flashed before me. When was the last time I told him I loved him? Could I remember the last time I tucked him in to sleep? When was the last time we laughed together?

Although I grew up learning the importance of love, kindness, and spending time together, until that day I never really appreciated the importance of those magical moments and the precious "last times" in life. He was still on the East Coast and I was home on the West Coast. After I called him to make sure he was okay, I held my two younger children, Oliver and Samantha, a little tighter while I thought about all the victims, their families, and the last times they were together.

Not only has 9/11 shaped our nation; it has shaped many of our lives. The gift for all of us in this tragedy is to cherish, remember, and hold dear the gift of our lives each day because tomorrow is promised to no one. There is magic in every breath, every moment, and every day. We just have to take the time to find it.

REFLECT

- If you knew it was the last time you would see a loved one, what would you say?
- What would you do?
- How would your experience with them change in the moment?
- We all know those last times will come, yet remembering that now, what would you like to experience now with the people you love?

We can't always see the gifts during a tragedy, yet there can be an empowering meaning that carries on to the next chapter of our lives. Anthony Robbins teaches, "There are no good or bad events in life, just the events and the meanings we give them." We may not always see the gifts, the magic, or the empowering meaning in the moment, yet those messages and meanings will come when the time is right. How would your life change if you remembered that there are gifts and lessons in every experience, even the most challenging ones?

The Ultimate Father-Son Moment – Randy's Story

In 1976, I was still in law school. One morning, during a constitutional law class, I was called to the dean's office for a phone call. The call had come from the cardiac floor of the hospital where I had taken my wife the night before for a checkup and an overnight stay. Without giving me any details, the station nurse advised me to come to the hospital as quickly as possible. My wife had suffered from a pulmonary embolism for several years, and I knew this call was not a good omen.

I picked up my in-laws, who happened to be visiting, and went to the hospital. When we arrived we were escorted to a windowless room and were told that my wife had passed out earlier that morning on the way to brush her teeth and had not yet regained con-

sciousness. We waited for what seemed like an eternity before her cardiologist came into the room. It was probably no more than ten minutes. He looked at us and simply said, "She's gone." She had thrown another clot, and it was more than her heart could tolerate. I cannot recall what transpired at the hospital after hearing the news because I was operating as if in a dense fog.

The next thing I remember is being back at my apartment trying to figure out what I was going to tell our six-year-old son. I drove to the school and made my way to his classroom. I briefly explained to his teacher what had happened and asked to take him home. I had never picked him up from school before. When he saw me standing in the doorway, a panicked look flashed across his face and then quickly disappeared.

We went to a local fast food joint and got plain cheeseburgers and French fries – his favorite. I found it impossible to grow impatient, as I usually did, with the extra time it took to prepare his special order. I suggested we eat outside where he could play if he wanted to. It was a sunny but chilly October afternoon. He played a little bit, chasing fall leaves as they blew in the breeze. We ate our meal and I asked him how his day had been and a dozen other similarly meaningless questions—just to put off for a few minutes more what I knew I had to say.

Finally, I pulled him onto my lap. I put my arms around him, almost as though I was trying to keep him, or me, from falling apart. I took a deep breath and told him that Mommy had gotten very sick that morning and would not be coming home – ever. She had gone to heaven where she wouldn't be sick anymore. He sat still for a moment or two and then leaned into me. He didn't sob, but I knew he was crying. I cried too.

We sat there for the longest time just feeling the crisp breeze and watching the leaves play in the sunlight. We bonded in the silence of the magical moment that afternoon – a meaningful and magical bond that has never been broken, even after the passage of more than thirty-five years.

Saying Goodbye

How lucky I am to have had someone in my life that made saying goodbye to them so hard....

– A.A. Milne, Winnie-the-Pooh

When life takes a child early, we can't help but feel the sorrow in such tragic moments. Yet through the experience, there can still be shining glimpses of grace, love, and meaning.

Free *– Ebo's Story*

I truly feel that magical moments happen to us every day. In July 2013, my son and I went to the Zac Brown concert with another mother and son, our best friends. To attend a concert with your teenage sons is a magical moment in its own right! But that July night was special. My friend Gini and I had been planning this night for months. Our sons, Nolan and Ebo, were very close friends who grew up playing ice hockey together. They both shared dreams of playing ice hockey in college and someday maybe in the NHL.

You see, in November of 2011, Ebo was hit with devastating news. He had been experiencing a lot of pain in his right knee and thought he had torn a ligament. He was a very talented ice hockey player. When he consulted an orthopedic surgeon he discovered the root of his pain was much worse than a torn ligament. He was told that he had osteosarcoma, a very deadly form of cancer. Ebo's road ahead would be long and difficult. He would endure twelve months of intensive chemotherapy, have a knee replace-

ment surgery, and have five inches of his femur removed to fight the cancer. Through his journey he stayed positive and was an inspiration to his family, friends, and especially my son Nolan. We celebrated the end of his treatment with a party in October 2012. It was a relief to have that grueling treatment behind him.

Then in April 2013, I received a text from Gini that simply said...

Ebo's last scan did not come back clear. He has 5 nodules on his lungs, 2 on his left – 3 on his right. There will be 2 separate surgeries to remove the tumors. The first surgery is this Tuesday. Then in two to three weeks he will have a second surgery. He did not want people to know until after the prom. We have known for over a week. His battle begins again... wanted to let you know :(

My heart skipped a beat and I became overwhelmed with emotions. I cried so much my eyes started to burn. As a mother, it is hard to watch such an amazing family and incredible child go through such a painful journey. Ebo had to endure yet another surgery. The cancer was back, and the mere thought of that was terrifying. Life for this wonderful young man did not seem fair. I realized that sometimes we take too much for granted.

One day Gini and I were talking, and we thought it would be fun to make special plans to do something that summer. We wanted to plan something that the boys could look forward to doing together. Nolan and Ebo both loved country music. When Ebo was spending days and nights in the hospital, he would listen to music for hours at a time, oftentimes with his mother by his side. Gini and Ebo fell in love with the Zac Brown Band. Attending a Zac Brown concert in July seemed like the perfect thing to do with the boys.

Ebo had his second surgery on May 1, 2013. We planned to go to the Zac Brown concert on July 21. The concert gave us something to think about other than his diagnosis. Unfortunately, just forty-one days later another scan revealed four more nodules. Ebo would have to endure yet another invasive surgery to remove more tumors. I prayed that Ebo would be healthy enough to enjoy the concert.

July 21 arrived and I was so grateful that Ebo was feeling up to a night out with family and good friends. It was raining so hard that an umbrella was useless. The kids did not seem to be bothered with the fact that it was pouring even though we were going to an outdoor concert. I found them amusing. We splurged and hired a limo for the boys, and it arrived early. The kids eagerly got into the limo and away we went. I think someone was looking out for us because the rain stopped shortly before we arrived and the sun peeked out from behind the clouds! The kids walked around and visited with friends. We met back at our seats when the concert began.

My favorite moment was watching the boys sing along with the Zac Brown Band. They were your typical teenage boys who knew every word to every song. One song in particular stood out in my mind. The song's title is "Free" and the words in the chorus are...

> *Just as free, free, as I'll ever be*
> *Just as free, free, as I'll ever be....*

When I looked at the boys, I realized that they were caught up in the moment. They were singing the lyrics, and they were arm in arm. They were smiling from ear to ear. They were truly enjoying the moment. They were truly free. It was magical.

Ebo was always happy and had never complained during his battle with cancer, but it was especially nice to see Ebo and his friends so happy that night. In that moment in time they were teenagers looking so carefree and happy. The Zac Brown Concert was one magical moment that I will carry with me and treasure forever.

Unfortunately Ebo lost his two-year battle with cancer on Christmas Day. He died peacefully in his mother's arms surrounded by his family. My son Nolan and I attended the funeral. Gini asked Nolan and ten other teenage friends to speak at Ebo's funeral. I was amazed that all eleven boys were able to speak with such love so clearly and share special memories about their dear friend. They loved Ebo so much. I knew how special Ebo was to Nolan. Nolan told Ebo's parents, Steve and Gini, that Ebo had always been an inspiration to him. He also told them that Ebo was his hero and that he will treasure the time he spent with him playing ice hockey and listening to country music. At the funeral, I had a flashback to July, and I was grateful for that magical moment we shared.

Ebo is free, as free as he will ever be. We love you, Ebo.

There is power in words. But you need to *be there* to hear and appreciate them. Being there is more than being physically present; it means being present in your attention, your heart, your soul, and your body. Many people can be physically present with you but not really present with you in their mind and spirit. We have all been with people who seem to be more focused on texting on their cell phone, reading something on their iPad, or working on their computer. Yet you have to be truly present, without all the distractions, to even come close to realizing it's a magical moment. It's in those truly present moments that grace and love will appear, even when you least expect it.

You Are Wonderful – *Melissa's Story*

My friend Melissa lives a big life – lots of travel, events, family, friends, and things to do. She is a loving mother, a devoted wife, and a dear friend to me. We have shared more magical moments and meaningful times together than I am able to count. She is one of those friends that you know would drop everything for you if you needed her. True-blue friends like Melissa are hard to come by and are a treasure in life. We have shared countless stories of life, challenge, love, hardship, and inspiration.

As the years pass, she just gives and gives more to her family. People count on her and she provides selflessly. Love is not just a verb for Melissa – it is her identity.

A few years ago, her father, Tom Parker, or for those who knew and loved him, "Geep," suffered a massive stroke that resulted in severe memory loss similar to dementia. Despite her very full and very busy life, she would go to see him frequently in the home where he was living. She would sit patiently with him and be the devoted daughter we all dream of having.

People suffering from memory loss can periodically have moments of lucidity. One afternoon, she and I were talking and she shared with me one such moment she had with her father. During one of her visits, her father looked into her eyes, held her hand, and said, "You are wonderful." Those were the last meaningful words her father spoke to her. Soon after that experience, her father passed away.

When she shared this with me, her whole body shifted and her countenance changed. I saw her light up with spirit, grace, and gratitude. Melissa has a lot to be proud of – her tireless work for numerous organizations, her successful and happy children, and a husband who is recognized for making meaningful change in the world through his profession – yet those three words from her father seemed to give her a gift and a magical moment that was a unique, meaningful, and true legacy for her to hold dear in her heart. Melissa, YOU are wonderful.

The Words "I Love You" Never Meant So Much –

Margaret's Story

My father was a war hero. We are from the Philippines, and he served in the US Army, doing his duty in World War II, the Korean War, and the Vietnam War. It was in Vietnam that he was unfortunately exposed to Agent Orange, and years later it manifested into cancer, which ultimately took his life.

During the painful days before he passed, I would spend time with him and enjoy his sense of humor and warm smile, and still learn the many lessons he had to share.

It wasn't within the Filipino culture in which my parents were raised to openly express emotions. One day when I was saying goodbye, I said, "I love you, Daddy," as I always did for years, whether in person or on the phone. His standard response was "Okay." But that one precious day, when I told him I loved him, he looked at me while lying in bed and said, "I love you too," and winked as he used to do. I never thought four words could mean so much, and I was engulfed with such love and emotion.

Tell someone today that you love them. Don't take for granted that they will always be there.

That moment will always be the most memorable of my life. My daddy will always be my hero. I love you back, Daddy. You are forever in my heart.

REFLECT

- Have you ever been with someone – a spouse, a child, or a friend – who was distracted by technology and not fully present with you? How did that feel?

- When was the last time you spent time with loved ones? Were you all truly present with each other?
- What would have to happen for you to disconnect from your modern life and truly be present with those you love?

Thanks for the Memories

Have you ever had a moment when you were trying to make the right decision and a memory of someone flashed in your mind and you instantly felt better and knew what to do? Have you ever paused and a past event flashed before your eyes and put a smile on your face?

Many of those memories are merely magical moments rising to the surface for you to capture and enjoy for the moment.

The Race – *A Moment with My Father*

I remember running by myself in the San Francisco Chronicle half marathon years ago. At one point in the race, I was running through the San Francisco Presidio and started feeling very tired. My legs were burning and begging me to stop. My breathing was heavy and strained. My pace was dragging. I was clearly hitting the wall. At one point, I turned on the street heading directly to the San Francisco Marina and was jolted by the beautiful sunshine just breaking through the clouds. At that moment, I felt an overwhelming love envelop me. My father had passed away many years earlier, but, in that moment, memory after memory of him raced through my mind – the joys, the sorrows, the fun, his illness, the moments being daddy's little pumpkin princess – all overtook me like a wave of energy. I realized that my father was with me. As tears streamed out of my eyes, I realized the magic in that moment. I was reliving moments that were long hidden in the attic of my memory. I didn't feel alone and I certainly didn't feel tired any longer. I realized that I hadn't had my last time with my father. He was with me again and is always with me. I sailed through the rest

of the race in my own private bliss. Wow – even remembering
those moments now, that race was truly one of the most amazing
wins for my body, my mind, and my spirit. Thanks for the memo-
ries, Daddy, and for all you continue to do to inspire me in life.

REFLECT

- Can you think of a time when you remembered someone
  or something in your past and it helped you through a
  challenging time?
- What was the magic in that moment?

Life's Passings

If I Had My Life to Live Over

by
Erma Bombeck

I would have talked less and listened more.
I would have invited friends over to dinner
even if the carpet was stained and the sofa faded.
I would have eaten the popcorn in the "good" living room
and worried much less about the dirt
when someone wanted to light a fire in the fireplace.
I would have taken the time to listen to my grandfather
ramble about his youth.
I would never have insisted the car windows be rolled up
on a summer day because my hair had just been teased and sprayed.
I would have burned the pink candle sculpted like a rose
before it melted in storage.
I would have sat on the lawn with my children
and not worried about grass stains.
I would have cried and laughed less while watching television
and more while watching life.

I would have shared more of the responsibility
carried by my husband.
I would have gone to bed when I was sick
instead of pretending the earth would go into a holding pattern
if I weren't there for the day.
I would never have bought anything just because it was practical,
wouldn't show soil, or was guaranteed to last a lifetime.
Instead of wishing away nine months of pregnancy,
I'd have cherished every moment and realized that
the wonderment growing inside me was the only chance in life
to assist God in a miracle.
When my kids kissed me impetuously, I would never have said,
"Later. Now go get washed up for dinner."
There would have been more "I love yous," more "I'm sorrys"...
but mostly, given another shot at life,
I would seize every minute...look at it and really see it...live it...
and never give it back.

In memory of Cindy Main (FA parent),
who lost her fight with cancer in January 1999.

Memories are powerful reminders of life. We can focus on the challenges and problems in someone's life or we can celebrate the beautiful times, the moments of laughter and happiness. We choose the meaning we give to all the lives around us, including our own.

REFLECT

- What meaning have you given to your relationship with people in your life who have passed on?
- What do your own life experiences mean as a result of having them in your life?
- What decision could you make to enjoy life more right now with the people in your life?

Last Dance – *A Father and Daughter Dance*

My father was a beautiful man. He loved his family, cherished his children, and overcame challenges with alcohol to become a brilliant ballroom dancer. I believe he gave up alcohol when he found his bliss in dancing.

I had the honor and privilege of dancing with my father at several ballroom events. When I hear the Luther Vandross song "Dancing with My Father," I can't help but feel a tear on my cheek—not from sadness, but from the immense joy those moments continue to give me. I searched the recesses of my mind and to this day still haven't been able to locate the memory of the last dance with my father. However, the search continues with great pleasure as I relive the moments where he would say, "Honey, wait for the floor to clear, I like to make an entrance" or "I need to go to the car and change my shirt; women like dancing with a man who wears a clean shirt" or "I need to wax my shoes so I can glide across the floor like Fred Astaire." He never remarried after his divorce with my mom and instead continued to be a bit eccentric, living in a small studio apartment and dating and dazzling women with his charms and footwork.

He came to me when he was seventy saying he needed to buy some Sergio Valenti jeans to keep up with the fashion, and he proudly wore his new jeans for some dance nights so he would look "hip." There were times he would come by my house first and I would gently wipe the hair dye off his cheek and neck. Due to his zealousness in being "hip," he would sometimes over dye his hair or over spray his men's cologne – smelling a lot like a French bordello.

When I was twenty-two, I ran a daycare center. My father would periodically come and play with the kids, dance with them, and make them laugh. I enjoyed seeing the bliss in his eyes, especially when he spent time with his grandson Justin.

All in all, I never heard my dad complain one time in his life. He would give you the shirt off his back if he felt you were cold, or the money in his bank account if he felt you needed it—even if it left him with nothing. He was giving and loving and truly loved my brother Richard and me.

Then one morning I received a call from the local hospital saying that my father had driven himself there the night before with chest pains. The nurse told me he refused to give my phone number to anyone because he didn't want to bother me since I worked so hard as a single mother and had a son to raise. They finally convinced him that it was critical. When they called they told me to hurry. I ran my baby son to a neighbor and jumped in my car, wiping the flood of tears from my eyes so I could see my way. I still remember the morning haze and the sun just starting to rise. When I arrived, the doctor sat me down and told me my dad wouldn't make it through the day. I immediately went to my father's side, kissed him gently, and told him how much I loved him and that he was such a blessing in my life. He smiled at me and held my hand. I could see the love in his eyes and feel the tenderness in his touch. Words really weren't necessary as we had a lifetime together.

Then the heart monitor alarmed, blue and red lights started flashing, and noises were all around me in a song I am sure the hospital hears every day. The nurses and doctors flew into the room and swept me away from his side, as I reached for him one last time. They pulled me into the waiting room and I sat there stunned and alone. The doctor came out shortly after and said my father had passed. He said it was remarkable that he lasted until I arrived. He really didn't think he would. I knew he would because he understood the power of last times, and I was his little pumpkin princess, and it didn't matter that I was an adult now – I always was his little girl and I always will be.

As I write these words, I feel that moment in my body – the intensity of love and the power of the last time I was with him on his last day in this life.

Legacies that pass from generation to generation last much more than a lifetime. If you take a moment to think about it, history is a recounting of lessons from generation to generation. The more intimate stories within families create a familial bond that illustrates the uniqueness of a family.

A Lesson of Generations from Oji-San –
My Grandfather's Garden

I was born in Japan and my family moved to the United States when I was quite young. We would go back to Japan every summer, however, and visit my grandparents in the family home. It is tradition in Japan that houses are passed down from generation to generation, and this house had been in our family for fourteen generations.

My grandfather was a senior vice president of finance for Matsushita Electric, now Panasonic. Always the corporate professional, he never took off from work but surprised me one day when I woke up and, sitting there smoking a cigarette, blowing smoke rings, was my grandfather. He said he had a special day planned for me that day. I would spend the day with "Oji-San," my grandfather. He was a thin, frail man, five-foot-seven, with a commanding, deep "Mr. Miyagi" voice.

I remember there was a different energy around the house that day. My mother and grandmother were in the kitchen preparing breakfast, and as I entered the kitchen I was feeling very awkward not knowing what was really going on this morning, so I asked them, "Okay, what's the deal?" My mother chuckled and responded that it was a special day to hang out with my Oji-San and do – yard work! – something I had seen him do religiously on the weekends. I was assured this was a different day and was instructed to go outside because he was waiting for me. At that time my mother handed me a very large container of warm gohan (rice): I had seen this rice before but was never quite sure what it was for. Little did I know I was about to find out.

As I approached my grandfather he was sitting by the pond, and I noticed he was talking to someone. I looked around and did not see anyone else around and soon realized that he was speaking to the koi. It was his hobby to breed this unique type of fish, which came in vibrant colors of gold, purple, blue, and red. He asked if I brought the gohan, which I soon learned was special rice for the fish. He was talking to the fish as we were feeding them gohan. And I must admit I felt very confused and inquisitive but did not want to interrupt my grandfather! I needed answers, so I told him I was thirsty and ran back to the kitchen to talk to my mother. I told her I thought he was going crazy because he was talking to the fish. She smiled and told me to go back out – with glasses of water in hand for both of us.

Meanwhile, back at the pond, Oji-San was telling the fish they were beautiful and thanking them for being there and blessing the space of the pond and creating relaxation for all of us. There were several ponds, so there were many beautiful koi to see and each had a very unique personality and presence within the ponds.

After finishing up with the koi, we went to the serenity garden, where he told me he would teach me the art of creating serenity in a space. He picked up a rake, thanked it for allowing him to use it, and started to create this beautiful pattern in the rocks. And now he was talking to the rocks! He told them, "I apologize for stepping on you. But you'll be beautiful when I'm done." This incited another visit to Mom in the kitchen, where I proceeded to tell her my grandfather was talking to the ROCKS now! She had tears in her eyes at this point and said something to my grand-mother in Japanese, then told me, "Oh, silly boy. Go back out."

Oji-San now had a bucket and was pulling weeds out along the perimeter of the rock garden. But he was not throwing them away. He placed them gingerly in the bucket and told me we were going to replant them in the side of the field of weeds adjacent to the property, because he was not going to kill these plants.

We then went to a grove of bonsai trees that he'd been trimming and replanting around the property. He raised them and gave them to friends and neighbors. It's a distinction and honor because it takes years to grow them. So he's taking the wire and he's talk-ing to the wire and he goes, "Ah, you're a strong wire. May you be strong and hold the tree in the right position." And as he's clip-ping the tree, he's saying, "I'm sorry" to the tree again. "I'm sorry, but trust me. Discomfort now will create more beauty as you continue to grow." Then he turns to me and says, "Okay, you work hard. Time for lunch." And I'm relieved: "Great, domo arigato gozaimasu [thank you so much for this time]." He goes, "We go get ice cream later." I said, "Great, Grandfather. That would be wonderful."

I went back in the house, and as I was talking to my mom she said, "Okay, let's sit down and talk about the events of the day." I said, "Thank you, because I don't know what's going on." She said, "Do you know why you feel so comfortable when you come to this ancestral home?" I said, "No, but it always feels really good." She continued, "It could be nine months, twelve months, between visits but it always feels like you're home, right? That's because your grandparents are Zen Buddhists, as was I before I converted to Catholicism. And we had always believed that everything has an energy. And that if you provide the right vessel that soul and energy will come back.

"When you fed the koi, you were feeding fourteen generations of family, friends, and noble spirits. When you created the pictures in the rock garden, you were creating a space for your ancestors. So all the people that have been loved and in your life reside at this home. And that energy still stays here. And that's the reason why your grandfather has bred the koi. He forms the trees to give them the most beauty possible so that the souls of all these people that have been here will stay here. And in that space, that's where you find the connection to your family, into that energy. Because your whole life is much more than just beautiful things. It's when you take beauty and appreciate it. And then link that to something that's meaningful in your life."

What I left out was that I made a smiley face in the rock garden while my grandfather was creating stunning patterns that were perfectly linear and symmetrical. The care he took of it left such an impression on me. And I noticed he didn't force anything. Everything was organic and effortless movement. Just natural. And so, he goes, "You try." He literally bowed, which he NEVER did, you know, to grandchildren. He bowed and handed me the rake. And I asked, "Can I do it in the middle?" He said, "Yes. How will you get to the middle?"

He had these boulders. So I started jumping from boulder to boulder until I got in the middle. And I drew a big smiley face. From where he was standing he couldn't really see it, and I could see he was trying to figure out how to get a better vantage point to see. He kind of tiptoed out on the boulders and stood in the middle. I'll never forget what he said: "Best picture ever." And he had a big smile on his face. He was grinning from ear to ear.

It was at that moment that we had that precious connection. And that was a lesson from when I was eight. Just talking about it gives me goose bumps...the energy of the memories that I will always hold dear for the rest of my life. Thank you, Oji-San.

Roxy's Magical Garden *– A Grandfather's Gift*

When I was very young, my grandparents sold their home to my parents so they could build their own dream home. I'll never forget the moment when my grandfather, whom we all lovingly called Baba, showed me blueprints of his custom home and asked me, "What do you think would make this the perfect home?" I told him that when the house was finished, I wanted a big rose garden like the one in Alice in Wonderland with a maze that you could get lost in for hours. Obviously, that seemed like a crazy request to everyone, but my grandfather saw it differently.

He told me that he wanted me to spend a lot of time at his home and he would make sure I had exactly what I wanted. Throughout the construction of their new home, my grandfather would drive me there and keep reminding me, "This is where your garden is going."

When the home was finished, I couldn't believe my eyes! In the exact place my grandfather showed me, there was a trellis with roses wrapped around it that led to a gravel maze with bushes growing all around it. He planted cucumbers and tomatoes that he promised would grow tall and hide the path. Sure enough, when I was a little girl, I was small enough to spend hours upon hours hiding behind bushes with my cousins and racing to the end of the maze. It was my dream come true.

When I was in middle school, I had some challenges dealing with a few tragic deaths in my family, and my parents thought I should meet with someone to help me cope with the loss. Luckily for me, my grandfather was not only a loving patriarch but also a practicing psychiatrist! When I outgrew hiding in the maze, spending time in the garden with my grandfather was still part of my weekly routine. We would spend countless hours trimming the roses, picking cucumbers and tomatoes, and maintaining the beautiful pathway he had built especially for me. During these times we would discuss my future, my relationship troubles, and my favorite hobbies and activities. He never made me feel like I was "in session"; he was more like my confidant and best friend. He was someone I could trust with any kind of information. He wouldn't just listen, he would also share stories of his past that would relate to my present and help me discover possibilities for my future.

When I discovered that he had been diagnosed with cancer, my world started spinning. Initially I became selfish and withdrew from my grandfather, worried that I couldn't hold myself together in front of this frail man that was always so strong. He had been secretly battling the disease for a few months because he didn't want to hurt or burden his family.

I finally came to my senses and decided I did not want to spend the last years I had with him focusing on the times I wouldn't have with him, but that I would rather appreciate the quality time I had with him while he was still with me. Whenever I could, I would take him to chemotherapy. Sometimes I would take my study material and just sit by his side when he was too exhausted to talk. Other times we would take snacks and turn the therapy into a picnic where again we acted like we were in the garden – just planting flowers and talking about matters both trivial and important.

I'll never forget asking him how the treatments were working. He just said he had the results sent to my uncle because, as long as he felt good, he didn't need to know how long he had to live. He reminded me that every moment he spent alive was to be cher-

ished with the memories he already had and the memories he was making with those around him.

When he passed, my family had to rent a large tent to house all the people that came to his memorial service. The funeral home wasn't big enough so we stood in the rain -- not even able to hear the service. Each person who came to pay their respects shared similar stories. Stories of the man he was to them and the love and respect he showed. I can say that those who were lucky enough to know him continue to be filled with memories and lessons from his long and meaningful life.

Just this past summer, my mother and I went to the nursery to buy plants for his garden, one that had been through a harsh winter and needed some TLC. As if nothing had changed, my mom and I spent hours laughing and reminiscing about my grandfather and talking about our past, present, and future together, there in the garden.

Baba left a legacy of joy when he passed away, and I will treasure those moments for a lifetime.

Baba, I will love you forever. Please know that you are shining sunlight on our magical garden each and every day. Each time I am there is a magical moment with you.

REFLECT

- What legacies and lessons have you learned from your ancestors?
- How do you honor their memory?
- What beliefs, values, experiences, and magical moments are you passing on to your children and grandchildren?

Heroes

Heroes come in all shapes and sizes. We all know different people who embody what we each believe to be heroic. Yet there are some universals where people face overwhelming odds and through it all truly personify what it means to be heroic through their courage, fearlessness, and integrity. Such role models bring each of us treasured magical moments that can lift us in life and show us a guiding light through life's twists and turns.

Here is a story about a young man who was truly a hero through overwhelming challenge.

Heroes Are Made in Clutch Time – *A Mother's Reflection*

WOW! What an infectious smile...a bright-eyed dazzling twinkle...melting the hearts of girls and bonding the souls of young men. That was Eric Eberling, affectionately known by his friends and family as "Ebo." So many magical moments throughout his life...

Blond flowing surfer hair, blue eyes that captured your heart and the admiration and respect of his peers – welcome to Ebo. He lived and breathed hockey, baseball, and surfing, learning to ice skate at three and growing up to earn his place on Comcast's elite Under-16 American hockey team – a hockey player, a dedicated student, a devoted friend, a loyal Philadelphia Flyer fan, and a kind son who was generous with his spirit and caring with his heart.

During one of his hockey seasons, he began feeling pain in his leg and was concerned that it might be an old injury resurfacing. Concerned about his ability to do his best for his team that season, he went to the doctor. The diagnosis of metastatic bone cancer stunned all of us and led Ebo on his two-year battle, some-

times thousands of miles away, that truly tested the motto "Do your best, never give up, come out a winner." As the months progressed, we watched our boy handle his health challenges with grace, strength, and amazing courage – sometimes much more than many of us.

"At first it was devastating," said Ebo. "But when you go through what I went through, you realize that there are definitely more important things in life." Soon after he was diagnosed with cancer he continued his love of hockey through putting on his ice skates again and coaching the Team Comcast 00 Peewee hockey team.

Ebo's words were his deeds. "He's always positive," said Anthony Amato, one of the players Ebo coached. "He never puts us down. He always motivates us to do the right thing."

During those two years, so many people rallied to support Ebo and the role model that he was for so many. There was a "Stay Strong Ebo – No One Fights Alone" T-shirt campaign with Ebo's hockey number "24," along with countless other deeds to honor his challenge with cancer.

Throughout each of his numerous surgeries and chemo treatments, Ebo remained true to his positive and grateful outlook on life. He even regularly checked in with people to make sure they were doing well through some of their own life challenges. Rarely did he complain to anyone – he stayed strong and lived his life to the fullest, smiling that radiant carefree teen smile as he drove down the street in his favorite blue Jeep Wrangler with his license plate "Ebo 24." In his heart, we believe he cherished turning that key each time he sat in the driver seat, simultaneously cherishing his life and all the people in it.

On Thanksgiving 2013, Ebo tweeted, "There is just too much to be thankful for today. There is no possible way I can put it all into 140 characters." Two weeks later, he got accepted into college.

The next month, when we knew Ebo's condition was progressing rapidly, we sent out texts to his friends. Our house became a revolving door with a basement FULL of kids who were not scared and who just LOVED Ebo and wanted to be there for him. We had tears, laughter, movies, pizza, and a ton of LOVE in our home! Others came as they heard the news, and Ebo loved seeing everyone. I don't think Ebo really grasped at the time that the end was near—what teenager would? Yet Ebo greeted everyone and was so excited to see all of them, even during times when he was weaker and less than energetic.

Christmas was Ebo's favorite holiday, and it was fitting that we held him gently as he said goodbye to us this last Christmas 2013. His friends still come over to give us gifts of "magical moments" with Ebo and hang out for the night, sit in his room, and rekindle memories. The rallying and special tributes to Ebo have been nonstop. His high school friends share their plans for their senior trip just to keep us up to date and in the loop of what Ebo would be doing during this most special senior year. They NEVER forget to include us, and that is the most special tribute to our son! Ebo rallied our family, Lenape High School, the hockey community, and the Mount Laurel community in so many ways.

What I wasn't expecting and what has touched my life so deeply are the magical moments that occurred during and after his passing. We always knew that Ebo was a truly special kid, yet as parents many of us feel that our own kids are special. Every moment for me with Ebo was special, but of course I am his mom. But to hear each and every account of how my son touched and changed so many lives was so amazing and surprisingly uplifting during our time of grief. As parents, you teach your child many lessons in life—be kind, do the right thing, think of others, do well in the world, work hard, and so on. In life, there are so many opportunities for the kids to hold true and "test" those lessons. Ebo truly had his test and really did embody those life lessons and stay true to their virtue throughout his seventeen years and during his battle with cancer. Now, after his passing, there is such magic in hearing more and more how our son genuinely touched lives. It's as if the swirl of Ebo's spirit continues to wrap his arms around others and us.

One student from Ebo's high school shared with us that he was afraid to go to an interview and then said, "Ebo wouldn't have been afraid."

Another friend told us of an awkward situation he was recently in and said, "What would Ebo do?"

His closest best friends confided to us that they live every day now thinking, "I want to do this for Ebo."

We continue time and time again to learn how much our son has touched other people's lives. Many parents are not ever given this gift, and to have these moments now is both heartbreaking and inspirational.

Ebo's magic in his life and his legacy in passing is an inspiration and gift to those of us who remember him. We love you, Ebo... thank you for being a guiding light to so many. My magical moments continue to come from you and from me being so proud to be your mom.

I feel your spirit and love reminding others and me to "Do your best, never give up, and come out a winner..."

REFLECT

- What does being a hero mean to you?
- Who are the heroes in your life?
- What magical moments have you had knowing those heroes?

Taking Time

Sometimes in the midst of our busy lives, we might find it challenging to have time for the people we love the most. One of the greatest gifts we can give someone is to "make" time for him or her even if we believe we don't "have" the time. At the end of our lives, I don't recall many people saying, "I wish I made more time for work, errands, the many to-do items on my lists, and endless other things that can take up a day." More often than not people wish they made more time for the people they love. Why not take time to have a magical moment with someone you love right now?

Taking a moment to be grateful is one of the most profound gifts you can give another person. Too often we let time pass thinking there is always another tomorrow. In the midst of our busy lives, many of us forget to live and be present. As the great lyrics from the song by Stephen Stills say, "Love the one you're with…."

Lessons of a Lifetime: A Daughter's Final Goodbye to Her Father – *Tammy's Story*

> *My dad was a pioneer ahead of his time. In the early seventies he was healing with energy, an uncommon medical practice of the era. He spent the last thirty years of his life dedicated to serving and healing people. I remember my dad's love for people; he touched many hearts throughout his lifetime. My dad had such an incredible mind that when he got dementia it was so strange to see that incredible mind drift away. As he got progressively worse, we*

ended up having to place him in a hospital. At one point, my dad lost fourteen pounds in fourteen days; it was painful and frightening to see. At the hospital, they knew he was nearing the end, so they asked him, "Wendell, what do you want, what can we do for you?"

He said, "I want to see my family."

Mother's Day was that coming Sunday, which made it feel even more emotional to the family. When the hospital called, my brother picked up my dad and took him home. Psychosis had set in and he was not at his best. It ended up being an emotionally exhausting day. When it was time to take my dad back to the hospital, I volunteered.

When we began driving, his eyes were shut and his head was hanging low. After a few minutes, I pulled over and stopped. I took a deep breath and shared with my dad the lessons he had taught me. I recalled him telling me that I should never judge anyone, because I could never judge anyone until I could walk a mile in his or her shoes, and I would never walk a mile in their shoes. I remembered his love for people and how I had modeled that in my life. I shared with him the impact of who he was as a man, how he had helped shape my life and the lives of many others.

I shared with him that I loved him so much. I watched as his eyes stayed shut and tears rolled down his face. I dropped my dad off at the hospital. The next night I received a call that he had passed. I am so grateful that I was able to share the impact he had on my life and the lives of others. I was able to tell him how much I loved him, and in that moment I knew he heard me.

REFLECT

- Imagine you are looking back at your entire life from infancy to old age.
- Who would you want to spend more time with?
- What would you want to say to them?
- Who are you grateful for?
- How did you express that gratitude?
- What would have to happen for you to do all of this now?

Lessons from Our Parents

We never really appreciate the things our parents did for us until we start doing the same for our children.

– Author Unknown

As a child I remember rolling my eyes when my parents started reciting the important things I should remember and telling me how to live my life. As I have lived my life over these last five decades, I look back now and think of all the times I heard my father's voice teaching me those lessons with love and care. There were so many times that what he said was so important it impacted my life. Now I am saying those same things to my children, watching them roll their eyes and smiling to myself knowing that at one point in their future they will hear my voice and hopefully smile too with fond memories and love.

Three Life Lessons – *A Father's Legacy*

Growing up, my father taught me three very important life lessons. First, he taught me, "The gift is the giving." Second, he taught me, "Tell your truth with love." Third, he taught me to "cherish magical moments." He seemed to always have time for my brother and me. When he was with us, he fully embraced the moment, from his pause when he dropped me off at elementary school waiting for my kiss on his cheek, to building forts with us in our backyard, and in later years napping with his grandson Justin on his chest. He never ceased to create fun with his friends – right up to his passing. In his life, he was a model for experiencing and appreciating magical moments, and he is fondly remembered for sharing that magic with others.

This book honors the legacy of his three lessons. Thank you for allowing me to share my gifts with you, tell my truth with love, and share some magic that will transform the way you experience, honor, and appreciate your own life and the lives of those around you.

REFLECT

- What lessons have you learned from your parents?
- How have you incorporated those lessons in your life?
- Have you taught those same lessons to your children?

10

CHAPTER TEN

The Magic in Serving Others

Man is remembered by his deeds.

– Knute Nelson

As we have explored throughout this book, magical moments can happen anywhere, anytime, and with anyone – with family and friends, in our times alone, and even with memories of those who have passed.

We can also create magic by serving others through our good deeds. Helping others and serving the greater good can help us have a more fulfilling life and give us a special sense of meaning. We all have something to contribute, whether it's a brief gesture of kindness or a project for large-scale challenges facing our world.

Dean Nelson, in his book *The Power of Serving Others*, writes, "One of the biggest transformations I observed was that, when people began to serve others, they saw how easy it was to start wherever they were, regardless of their circumstances and resources. We don't have to go to different parts of the world to serve. We can serve the person we encounter next."

By taking the time to serve others, we can create magical moments that will have long-lasting positive effects on our world.

The Gift of Giving

The ultimate aim of the quest must be neither release nor ecstasy for oneself, but the wisdom and power to serve others.

– Joseph Campbell

Many people crave and seek happiness for themselves and fulfill this desire by giving to others. As Richelle E. Goodrich, author of *Smile Anyway*, has said, "We hunger after the sweet nectar of happiness without understanding that it is harvested from the flowering field of good deeds."

- Do you know someone who gives to others selflessly?
- Try to recall a time they have given to you. How could you emulate their selflessness?
- Can you remember the last time you gave to someone purely out of the goodness in your heart?

The Gift of Our Time

Time has a way of showing us what really matters.

– Margaret Peters

"I don't have enough time" is a phrase all too common in our fast-paced society. Our time has become one of our most valuable assets, and people crave more time to do the things they believe they need to make them happy.

In her article "Giving the Gift of Our Time to Others," written for the Stanford Graduate School of Business Center for Social Innovation, Marguerite Rigoglioso explores the concept of giving our time – even when most of us feel that we are constantly time constrained. She cites research that shows how "helping other people can actually increase feelings of 'time affluence' and alleviate the perceived 'time famine.' The research demonstrates that spending time on others makes people feel like they have done a lot with their time – and the more they feel they have done with their time, the more time they will feel they have."

Even when we don't think we have the time to make a difference we can open ourselves to others, and through little acts of kindness we can create magical moments. As Rabbi Harold Kushner so eloquently states in his book *Living a Life That Matters*, "We don't have to find the cure to cancer to make a difference to the world… we only have to share our lives with other people."

Go Now! – *A Son's Story*

What's in a moment? Time passing by, seconds, minutes, a day, a month, or a year? Routines…

7:43 a.m. – I make the call to my mom who is in the hospital for a stomachache. It mustn't take too long as I have to get my laptop running, prepare the reading assignments on the whiteboard, and get myself mentally ready to teach in twenty-seven minutes. The students will be here…soon.

"It might be cancer," she says. Silence.

"What? I thought it was a stomachache." My heart is racing. My mom might have cancer? I am suddenly overtaken with fear and stress. What to do? Call my wife, Gina.

I am fighting tears, and my throat is tight.

I tell myself to stay calm, be strong, and not cry. Why in fact is crying off limits? Turns out that it's not as I will shed many tears on this day and the ones that are to come.

I call Gina and say, "It might be cancer…"

"What!? I'm coming home! Leave school. Go to your mom right now! GO NOW!"

I pause. There are thirty-three students showing up any second. I call the school office secretary and say, "Hi, it's Mr. Kloes." My throat tightens and I continue, "My mom is in the hospital. I have to go."

"Go now" is all I hear on the other end. By now students have come into the room. They look at me and I look back at them. Silence…they know something is seriously wrong with Mr. Kloes.

"Go now." I leave, fast. I have no memory of the ride other than that it was sunny and it felt a bit odd to be somewhere other than my classroom several minutes after eight o'clock on a Thursday morning.

I get to the hospital and take an elevator to her room. My mom is lying in the hospital bed. No one ever looks good lying in a hospital bed.

My mom looks up and says, "What are you doing here?"

"Mom, where else could I be?"

"You didn't have to do that." Typical. Mom makes it out to be no big deal. Her attempt at the "everything is going to be just fine" attitude.

For lack of a better question, "How are you feeling?" comes to mind.

"Oh…fine. I am just waiting for some tests…the doctor should be here in a while."

A few moments later the nurse comes in and says, "Good morning, Mrs. Kloes, we have to get you ready for surgery."

My mom looks at me and I look at her. We are both stunned. Absolute shock and bewilderment.

"What surgery? Are you sure?" my mom gets out. "I don't know anything about this."

The nurse looks at the chart. "Yes, Mrs. Kloes, you are going into surgery in fifteen minutes. The doctor has determined that surgery must happen right now. Your son can step out of the room so we can get you prepped. He can come back in a few minutes and walk with you down to surgery."

As I sit here writing this story, I cannot for the life of me remember those minutes. Shock has a funny way of deleting what the brain cannot comprehend. From a stomachache to colon cancer in thirty minutes.

A moment later, "Mr. Kloes," the nurse says, "you can come back in."

By now my mom is wired up. "Call your dad...he'll want to know."

I call his number and wait for my dad to pick up. "Dad? Mom's going in for emergency surgery." I somehow get the words out even though my brain is moving way too fast. Surreal is the only word to describe the whirlwind that surrounds me.

"What? Now?"

"Dad, I'm walking her down right now."

I will never forget the look on my mom's face in that moment. Fear but also a determination. She says, "Well, if they have to do it, we may as well do it now."

But also, "Is your dad coming?"

All I can say is "Yes, he's coming."

What's in a moment?

I lock eyes with my mom's, hold her hand, and reassure her – and myself – that everything is going to be okay.

In that instant of time, in those precious seconds, I could have been in my classroom teaching. I would have been with thirty-three of my students, worried sick about my mom, but thinking that she was simply waiting on tests.

In those same seconds, she would have been alone to face one of the most dreadful experiences of her life.

In that moment of time, I was there to support her. My mind was swirling, gripped by the incomprehensible fear that my mom might be taken away, but at least I was there.

In that moment of time, those 108 seconds before she slipped behind the double doors marked "Surgery," I also saw a strength in my mom that I had never seen. I saw a toughness that looked the terrible situation in the face and said, "I will beat you."

It is amazing that in one of the most emotional moments of my life, I learned something about my mom that I had never before experienced.

The doors closed and the waiting game began. Time filled with phone calls, tears, fear, and hope.

As with so many moments in the last five years, my wife once again saw the situation clearly. "Go now." The cliché is that moments are fleeting. Indeed they are, but they also can leave a powerful impact on the moments that are to come, those seconds just around the bend, and those a little further off.

I learned an important lesson, or perhaps was reminded of one that happens time and time again. Priority must go to those you love. Magical moments happen when we realize time is a gift and it is precious. Take time for those you love and make time for the things that really matter.

REFLECT

- Think of someone from your past or in your life now who has made a huge difference.
- Have you ever taken the time to let them know?
- When was the last time you made time to visit them?
- Take a few minutes right now to find them. Then send them an email, call them, leave a voicemail, text them or write a letter.
- Gratitude is a beautiful gift in our lives, and giving it to those who have served us in life allows us to share our gifts.

Serving Those Less Fortunate

Every time you do a good deed you shine the light a little farther into the dark. And the thing is, when you're gone that light is going to keep shining on, pushing the shadows back.

– Charles de Lint

Many of us are fortunate to live very privileged and abundant lives. In the swirl of our hectic days, modern technology, and busy schedules, we often say we would like to do something "charitable" someday, yet for many of us that time is still far off in the future. The opportunities to do a kind deed, perform a selfless act, or give a moment of love are abundant in our lives. We just need to take a moment to notice them.

The Midnight Mission – *Oliver's Story*

I didn't know that two blocks could make such a difference in the life of a neighborhood. I was on my way with my mom and my sister to the Midnight Mission Center in downtown Los Angeles. I was driving through what looked like a very nice neighborhood, with families walking down the streets and couples eating at fancy restaurants. Then two blocks went by and everything changed. I saw streets filled with poverty. The sidewalks were filled with homeless people making shelters out of trash and cardboard boxes. People were walking with grocery carts full of whatever food they could find, and some were wrapped in dirty, old clothing just to stay warm at night. It was one of the worst neighborhoods I have ever seen in my life. I actually was a little scared as I drove down the street.

I remember seeing one woman whose image stayed in my mind. She looked about fifty years old. She was by herself and lived in an open cardboard box with a jacket on the top to keep in some sort of warmth. She was just sitting there looking blankly at the cars going by. I could see how hopeless she felt. Her eyes were dead, no happiness or hope was left in her. This had a very strong effect on me; I had no idea how bad it was in this area. As I pulled in to the Midnight Mission parking area, I finally felt safe, but I now knew that this neighborhood was a reality; these people actually had to live on the streets and find shelter day in and day out. I was here to help these people for just one day.

I walked in and was greeted by a friendly man who directed me to my station. I cooked and prepared food for the homeless population who visited the shelter. The man I was working with told me that all the workers in the facility actually live there and have been on the streets before. This amazed me because he looked like a clean-cut businessman. He said the center really helps people rehab back into normal life and get a job. I then prepared myself for the crowd about to walk in the door for food. As the line started forming, I was shocked by the situations some of these people seemed to be in. Most of them were drug addicts or alcoholics, and others were clearly suffering from severe mental illness. Even through all of those challenges, many were so immensely grateful and thanked me over and over again for serving them. I could see the look in their eyes and knew that they really appreciated the food and shelter they were given – even if it was only for a temporary moment. I felt like I was really giving back to the community and helping people that were in troubled situations.

After I finished, I paused and noticed that I felt changed. I saw how bad life can be if you make wrong choices. I learned that over one-third of the homeless population on Skid Row were college educated. Many have families. Many are recently unemployed. Many just fell on hard times. I committed to coming back and volunteering more of my time. There was more to be done, more people to help. I did go back a few weeks later and will be going back whenever I can to help. Meeting and interacting with the people in the shelter showed me that I have to be grateful for what I have every day and to not take life for granted. The homeless who came through for those dinners were very grateful for what they had, even if it was just a hot meal and a safe place to sit down for an hour.

The decisions you make in life can drastically change the outcome of your future. In just two blocks, you see the difference of lifestyles between people who are affluent and abundant, and those who are homeless with seemingly nothing. I will always be grateful for my life and the magical moments I experienced while volunteering at the Midnight Mission.

Breaking the Surface – *Julia's Story*

> *One of the most magical moments I have experienced was when I was teaching homeless and at-risk children from Los Angeles how to swim. Some of the children had never even seen a pool before. The fear in their eyes was strong as soon as they saw the water, and some of the children even refused to put their toes in. However, with the help of lifeguards and volunteers, all of the children eventually got in the pool. Smiles were shining so bright as they realized that they could overcome their fears! By the end of the week, the children who were originally scared to get in the water were jumping full force off the high dive! I will never forget the magical smiles that appeared once they realized the abilities that they thought never existed.*

REFLECT

- How do you contribute to your local community and the greater good?
- What can you do to serve others who are in need right now?
- How would that make you feel?
- Who inspires you in your life by being a shining example of doing good in this world?

Do the Right Thing

Have you ever had someone in life just give you a break? Sometimes a magical moment can spring from that moment you "made a wrong turn" and someone takes the time to set you back on course. Those memories can multiply exponentially in life when you too have the opportunity to give someone a break and help them get back on track.

Writing in Cement – Actions and Consequences

My husband is a sergeant with the Chicago Police Department. What is unique about my husband is that he invested in himself and got training to really help people. For instance, when he sees someone in need with a sign near the expressway entrance, he doesn't shout at him or her "Hey! Get lost." He will get out of his patrol car and spend time with them to help them remember their resources.

One of my favorite stories about him was when he was parked in his patrol car near a house where contractors had recently poured cement. While he watched, a group of kids came up and started writing in cement. He got out of his patrol car and caught three of them. Eventually the others came back to the scene. He captured their information and then sat down with them one on one, and then as a group, and asked about their lives, their actions, and their consequences. He ended up making a deal with them.

He said, "I will make a deal with you. I will come back in twenty-four hours. If the cement is like new, I will not take you all in."

They all started collaborating. "Hey! I know someone who has cement." Or "I will help buy it!" Three others were standing out-side the circle with their arms folded. My husband approached them. "What are you guys going to do?"

They shrugged their shoulders and said, "What can we do?"

"Well, I'll tell you this," my husband stated, "if I come back in twenty-four hours and someone else has written in the cement, you are all going in."

"Ohhhh," they proclaimed. "It looks like we are guarding the cement then."

I was so anxious to find out the next day what had happened. I was so hopeful. When he returned from his shift, he told me the cement was like new. He had helped those children to understand conse-quences and he truly served them. When I asked my husband to share this story, he said, "Honey, you share this story; it's your magical moment."

Isn't it interesting how we find magic in other people's moments?

REFLECT

- Have you ever been given a break?
- What was the lesson, the gift, and the magic in you receiving this gift?
- Have you ever given someone else a break to serve them for their future?

Loving All Living Things

When we learn to love all living things,
we will learn to love all humanity.

– Author Unknown

We share this earth with an abundance of living things, including our animal kingdom. Through the busy hectic lives we lead, it is some-times challenging to remember that these animals are not only our neighbors, but for many of us they are important parts of our lives, giving us unconditional love, loyalty, and friendship. Learning to live in harmony with our animal kingdom is one of the greatest gifts we can give our world.

Rescuing Max – *A Cat's Journey to His Loving Home*

I think everything in life happens for a reason. In 2006, I was driving my son to school. I had seven children in my Expedition, and I was dropping them off at school early. On the way out of our development, something caught my eye. I saw this white tattered and fluffy ball of fur. I could not tell if it was a cat or a dog so I slowed down to take a closer look. Upon closer inspection, I realized that what I saw was a white Persian cat. It seemed a little odd to see a Persian cat outside. It didn't seem right.

I talked about that cat the entire way to school. I asked the children a million questions about the cat. When I dropped the kids off at Whitman Elementary, my son Nolan looked at me and said, "I know you are going back for that cat." He was right. I raced back to the development to find the cat fending off two dogs. I jumped out of my car and chased the dogs away. I realized that the cat was sick and severely malnourished. I immediately called two girlfriends to enlist their help in capturing the cat. We couldn't catch the cat, so we called animal control. We chased that cat for over an hour. He was scared. I was relieved when animal control finally caught him. We quickly learned that sending this animal back with animal control would probably result in him being euthanized. We had already named him Marsh. He had small twigs stuck in his fur. He was a mess.

I had spent half my morning rescuing him, and something told me not to turn him over to animal control. My friend's veterinarian took in stray animals, so we decided to take him there. I had to wait for two hours until they opened. We put Marsh in a large crate with lots of cozy blankets. He buried himself in the blankets and seemed content.

When the vet opened, I signed a lot of paperwork. The last question I answered was "We will do everything in our power to locate the animal's owners. If the owners are not located, will you adopt this animal?" I froze. I was only trying to help him out. I wasn't looking to adopt an animal. I answered the question "yes."

Two days later I received a call from the vet. No one was looking for Marsh within a hundred-mile radius. They asked me again if I was willing to adopt him and I asked if I could stop by to visit him. She also said that everyone in the office had fallen in love with him and it would be no problem finding him a home.

When I walked into the room where Marsh was being kept, the vet tech asked me if the cat knew me. I told her we only had a brief encounter the other day when I rescued him. She said, "Well, he certainly knows who you are." I looked into the cage and Marsh was standing at the front of the cage waiting for me. He was purring loudly. He recognized me. The vet tech said that she had been with him for two days and his reaction to me was different. He was excited to see me. I spent some time with Marsh and signed the final papers for adoption. I already had another cat. I was not in the market to adopt another pet, but Marsh was special. I felt he was meant to be a part of my family.

We brought Marsh home four days later, and my kids immediately renamed him Max. He was still severely underweight and his eyes were badly infected. He lived in my bathroom linen closet for three weeks. He would burrow in my linens. We were introducing Max to our cat Patches. She was eight years old and enjoyed being the only cat. We had a slight problem. Patches hated Max. She would make these horrible sounds whenever she sensed Max's presence. Max was patient. You could tell that he was so grateful to have a clean dry place to live with lots of food and love.

Three weeks after Max was adopted I took Patches to the vet for a routine teeth cleaning. It was the fourth time she had had her teeth cleaned. I didn't think anything of it. I received a call from the vet four hours after I dropped her off. She told me that Patches had died under anesthesia. My kids were devastated. It was really the first time my boys had experienced a loss. We brought the kids to the vet to say goodbye. I remember my son Johnny sobbing so hard that tears were streaming from his face. It was heartbreaking.

When we returned home Max walked into the room and jumped up on the couch between my boys. They sat and talked about how much they loved Patches. I looked over, and they were petting Max and telling stories. Max brought them comfort. I couldn't believe that I had stumbled upon Max on the way to school. I only drove the kids once a week because we were in a car pool. That day I was meant to drive the kids. I was meant to find Max.

I truly believe that everything in life happens for a reason. When people ask me if we rescued Max, I tell them that he really rescued us.

REFLECT

- How do you honor and respect the living things in our world?
- When was the last time you noticed the beauty of an animal in this world?

Simple Acts of Kindness

Be compassionate. And take responsibility for each other. If we only learned those lessons, this world would be so much better a place.

– Morrie Schwartz

Keep the Change – *A Story of Simple Kindness*

At breakfast before the workshop began, a young man was eating with a friend. During breakfast, the young man noticed an article on the front of the newspaper that he knew the speaker at the workshop would enjoy. When paying for his breakfast, he purchased the paper to give to the speaker. On his way out the door, he noticed a homeless man and gave him the change leftover from his purchases.

At the workshop, the young man gave the speaker the newspaper. The young man's friend and breakfast guest was truly touched and inspired by the young man's actions that morning. My husband happened to be sitting next to the friend who shared the story of what happened that morning. He explained that these simple acts genuinely moved him. Upon hearing the story, my husband was also touched by the young man's simple and kind gestures.

The workshop ended, and the next day it was time to fly home. Upon arrival my husband took the car to refuel. While standing at the pumps, a man approached him and asked him for money for food. My husband thought of the young man's story from the previous day. So when done filling the car with gas, he invited the man to eat at the restaurant next door. They sat and enjoyed lunch, and my husband took a genuine interest in asking about his life. What was his story? What had caused him to be where he was? What resources did he have that he had not noticed?

Little did that young man know that when he spared his change, his gesture would impact and serve another person miles and miles from home.

Everyday Gifts

My father had many challenges in his life, and through all those challenges he taught me a wonderful lesson. He used to say that when you are feeling low, do something kind for a friend or make new friends and do something kind for them. Even in those rare moments when you still might not feel great, when you engage in small acts of kindness, you give joy to someone else while you simultaneously feel it within yourself. We need not wait for a low moment to do something kind. Why not do it every day? I recently started a daily tradition called my *everyday gift*. Each day I remind myself to do something kind for someone. Even if it is merely sending a quick email to an old friend to send him or her my love, or smiling at a stranger on the street – the act of giving will inspire you for the rest of the day and possibly your whole life. What everyday gifts can you share?

The Toll – *A Family Drive*

> We were on our annual family trip to the mountains, and those long drives often gave us the chance to share magical moments and reflect on our year while we had a moment to pause. As we drove we were thinking of good deeds we had done and more that we could do together. As we waited in line to pay our toll for the bridge, one of our kids said, "Let's pay the toll for the people behind us! We will be the friends they will never meet!" As we passed the money to the toll taker, we said, "Here is our toll and the toll for the next two cars." He smiled as we drove off. Of course, the kids turned around in their seats to see the reactions, and my husband drove slowly so those two cars could pass us. We got honks and waves from both cars. A passing moment, brief smiles, and a momentary exchange of friendship and giving – life is good.

By taking time out to be kind to others, we will only spread happiness into the world. A simple act of kindness can be the first steppingstone in the bridge to many wonderful friendships. What act of kindness will you share today?

REFLECT

- What simple acts of kindness do you put out into the world?
- What can you do every day to give to others?
- What tradition does your family uphold that helps others?

Inspiration

You don't do kind deeds expecting kindness in return.
You don't do kind deeds because you deem the recipient worthy.
You do kind deeds because it's who you are, and because you
understand the powerful difference your gentle hand makes
in this dreary world.

– Richelle E. Goodrich

PK's Spin Class – Workout to Fill Your Body, Mind, and Spirit

It was five days before Christmas. I was leaving my house early in the morning with a friend to do some last-minute shopping for the holidays. As I ran down the stairs I said to myself, "I don't need to turn on the lights; it's a waste of electricity. I've gone down these stairs hundreds of times."

The next thing I knew, I was freefalling and crash landing on the tile floor in my foyer. Pain shot through my legs and arms. I couldn't even crawl to the door to alert my friend Sam, who was waiting for me in her car at the curb in front of my house. Pain was searing through my legs. I just lay there with tears flowing out of my eyes.

"Honey, are you okay?" My husband's voice was such a blessing as he came running down the stairs.

As he covered me with blankets and called out to my friend, I heard him say, "I heard the crash and knew something was wrong." Now my tears turned to sobs. Ambulance? Emergency room? I could hear them talking. Next thing I knew I was being lifted into Sam's car and swept off to the ER.

Over the next couple of months, my ankle and leg injuries kept me from moving much. I am normally a very active woman. I'm a mom, a wife, an entrepreneur, and I teach in ways that serve the greater good and help people live their most inspired life. All of these things make me really happy and keep me on the move most of my day. Much of that stopped while I healed. Those months were an interesting pause for me. Slowly during those months the restlessness I felt really affected my spirit. I longed for a way to move again, to feel my spirit lifted again, and to be back in my world again.

My physical therapist finally gave me the go-ahead and told me I could ride a stationary bike to rebuild the muscle in my leg. I went to the gym and started slowly. After a few weeks, I remembered that my gym had spin classes so I went to one.

What I received in that class was more than just exercise. There was magic in that room. The instructor, Philip Kessel or "PK" as his students lovingly call him, had and continues to have a true gift for inspiring each of us in our own way. I watched, listened, and moved on that spin bike as he gave his full being to us in the class. From the music he chose to the words he used, and the energy he exuded in the room, I felt my entire body, mind, and spirit lifted. PK has a way of sharing gifts with his students that are beyond exercise. People leave his class feeling energized, inspired, and invigorated. It is no wonder there are lines of people waiting to get into his class. For some of his classes you even need to sign up online a day in advance!

Some teachers have that innate ability to convey their message with their whole body, their whole essence, and their whole spirit. It's not just what they teach; it is who they are.

I continue to go to PK's classes and frankly have never had such an enriching experience with exercise. My magical moment was found on that bike, in that energized and inspiring room, and I was able to get back into the life I loved with my body, mind, and spirit totally renewed. I continue to have many more magical moments in PK's class and outdoors where I have a newfound love affair with my road bike and cycling in nature once again.

Thank you, PK, for the gift you bring to your students and their lives...especially me.

REFLECT

- Who inspires you in your life?
- Who do you inspire by being an example of inspiration and love?
- How can you find harmony and balance in your body, mind, and spirit?
- What everyday gifts can you give to others?

Let's make serving others a priority in our lives. Although we may not feel that we have the time or resources to really help anyone else out, we do. While it would be wonderful to dedicate weeks to building schools in third-world countries, or to donate large amounts of money to charities we support, we can also make a difference just by giving an hour of our time at a local shelter or donating our used clothing. We could also just start smiling more, or make an effort to hold open doors for people, or make sure we answer the phone when our friends call for advice. There are so many ways for us to serve others and contribute to the greater good. By giving to others we make the world a better place, and we create magical moments in the lives of others as well as for ourselves.

Cherishing the Moments

Life is merely a series of amazing moments. With each moment comes a fantastic and exciting opportunity to improve your life and the lives of others. So many of us let the moments pass, failing to take full advantage of each of these meaningful occasions. Like snowflakes from the sky, each moment is unique to itself, and no other will be exactly the same. With each passing moment, a celebration occurs. Linking these celebrations to these moments is what elevates those around you. As the moments are seized, happiness begins to flood into your life and truly covers you and your heart with warmth and joy.

If we shift the collective attitude to one centered on turning each snowflake into a snowman, the moments will continue to grow and expand to the point of becoming driving forces in your life. Just like a snowman, all the small moments come together to form something even bigger and more meaningful. Through celebrating the moments, you will lead with happiness and joy, and the warmth will radiate and the glow will fill the room. People will be drawn to you, and you will find that the "we" will be improved. Together we have focused our efforts on pointing you toward some of the most significant areas of your life where magical moments reside.

Magical moments live within your personal life and professional one, through your friends and family members, when you experience time alone and when you are surrounded by nature. They can be captured, reminisced, and relived. They stay with you forever and are always a point of reference and a reminder of all you have. But more than anything, they should be noticed and celebrated. They should be placed on a pedestal and elevated to a significant priority within your life.

In the celebrated play *Peter Pan*, J.M. Barrie writes, "The moment you doubt whether you can fly, you cease for ever to be able to do it." Magical moments are everywhere. They can be missed with a simple blink of the eye. Notice them; enjoy them; celebrate them. But most importantly, believe in them. Believe you deserve them and trust that they are yours for the taking. It is not just about knowing they exist, it is about believing you can connect with them. The moment you doubt them, you will begin to miss them. Every moment is simply an opportunity to nurture your heart, warm your soul, and elevate your happiness. I believe in magical moments. In fact, I live my life for them. And I am hopeful that through this book and through these words you have gained even more strength and are more able to believe in these magical moments.

You have the ability to fly – to use these moments as your wings and gracefully and freely navigate the open air. The more magical moments you experience, the higher you can soar and the quicker you can fly. Use these moments to give you the magic to fly. And don't look back. Seize the occasion to inject unprecedented happiness into your life and the lives of others. Celebrate the magic that each moment offers. Together, these magical moments are ours.

Gina Kloes

Passion…Energy…Love

Gina embodies all three. Her success comes from her passion and commitment to serve the greater good. Her word is her bond and, with Gina, what you see is what you get!

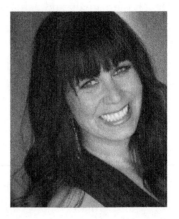

Educating People to Live the Life of Their Dreams…

Prior corporate lawyer and CFO, Gina Kloes is an inspired entrepreneur, author, corporate speaker and peak performance leadership coach, as well as a wife, mother, and artist. This book fuels Gina's mission to educate people through her "Magical Moment" initiative. This global movement inspires, educates, connects and supports individuals in their quest to live and embrace healthy and happy lives filled with more meaning, presence and engagement.

Gina's brand platform, www.ginakloes.com, is a place where mission-driven individuals, leaders and entrepreneurs can connect and recharge. In addition to offering retreats, leadership coaching and a variety of wellness programs, Gina also speaks on leadership, mindfulness, inspiration, entrepreneurship, financial freedom and of course, living a luscious life. She inspires people to live the life of their dreams while finding the true balance between their demanding, fast-paced, technologically focused lives and the joy and grace in pausing to appreciate the magical moments in life.

Over her twenty-five years of experience, she has successfully coached thousands of people from all walks of life on a wide range of life challenges related to health, relationships, family, to wealth, careers and business. She has helped people make their own successful choices to reach their goals and achieve their own personal sense of confidence, abundance, joy, and fulfillment.

Gina is a Vedic Master and certified instructor for the Chopra Center (founded by Deepak Chopra, MD, a global leader and pioneer in the field of mind-body medicine) teaching meditation, yoga and wellness. She is an instructor for Draper University of Heroes (founded by Silicon Valley icon, Tim Draper) an internationally recognized school for leadership and entrepreneurs from around the world. She has been the lead facilitator for the Anthony Robbins Foundation Making Strides Program. Gina is also a certified practitioner in the areas of Neurolinguistics (NLP) and time-line therapy.

To feel calm and peace right now, check out Gina's simple 21-day video and audio program for stress relief, *A Moment to Just Be*.

Making the World a Better Place....

Gina has designed several leadership and specialty programs for non-profit organizations serving the homeless and other challenged communities. She has taught at colleges, community groups, and high schools and middle schools on topics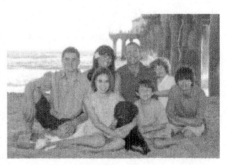

related to creating healthy personal relationships, identifying abuse, and ending domestic violence. She was featured on the Lifetime Cable Channel show *Motherworks*. She and her family regularly spend time volunteering at various homeless shelters and other organizations serving the greater good.

Behind the Scenes…

Gina has also coached a high school tennis team to win the championship in their region, cycled in many countries around the world, and completed numerous triathlons. She loves the ocean, and you can see her on many days swimming near the dolphins in the surf near her home. Her true inspiration comes from her loving family and their many friends and the magical moments they continue to create and share together.

To learn about Gina's retreats, programs and to book her to speak at your next event, go to www.ginakloes.com.

ABOUT THE MAGICAL MOMENT STORY CONTRIBUTORS

Julia Bakerink – Julia is a Broadcast and Digital Journalism major and Cinematic Arts minor at the University of Southern California. She recently worked with Dateline NBC and the KNBC Investigative Unit in Los Angeles. She is dedicated to the greater good through her work at *A Chance for Children*. As this book is published, Julia is about to studying in London for five months, where she will be taking journalism classes and exploring Europe.

Deborah Battersby – Deborah is a Chicago based Strategic Change Expert. She loves to challenge the status quo and works with entrepreneurs and executives around the globe to take their businesses to heights previously unrealized.

Suzanne Burns – Suzanne calls England home while she travels the world sharing her wisdom about health, energy and vibrancy through her extensive knowledge of the body, mind and spirit. Her deeper joy comes from her family, her friends and her pets who put a smile on her face and remind her everyday about what she values most in her life!

Vicki Bisset – Vicki's 15-year career in finance and investment banking in Australia, the UK and New Zealand led her to being the CEO of a top property development company in Tasmania. She works with investors and individual clients to remove the barriers to their success in lending and property ownership. Her exceptional skills as a personal development trainer are evident through her effective sales and human resources training worldwide in the business arena.

Scott Day – During the day, Scott is a National professional Small Business Coach. His passion for sports also led Scott to becoming a professional referee for college and high school football & basketball. Originally from Wisconsin, he now lives in Arizona and still plays golf in 100+ degree weather.

Gini Eberling – Gini's beauty and grace radiates through her love for all who touch her life. She continues to lift her husband, children, family and friends through showing them the gift and the gratitude in every moment of their lives.

Kevin Erdman – Kevin spends his time wrestling with his two kids Charlie and Sofia and dreaming of traveling Europe with his wife Valerie. As Creative Director for FOUNDER.org, a company-building program for student entrepreneurs, he lives his motto, "The best part of life is being of service to others."

Ashley Good – Ashley is a lover, mother, wanderlust and nomad. As a transpersonal coach and facilitator of personal brilliance, she is dedicated to the pursuit of truth and the practice of integrity, inspired by the conscious creation and cultivation of abundance and guided by grace, good vibes and the ripple effect of right action. Ashley whole-heartedly lives by the mantra that "Life isn't measured by the breaths we take, but the (magical) moments that take our breath away."

Lyn Hand – Lyn is a beautiful Aussie whose wisdom, intuition, and passion are evident in the people she serves as a highly respected psychologist, trainer for a well-respected personal development organization, and a woman who cares deeply for others. Her devotion to her family and friends is a true inspiration to all those who are fortunate enough to be in Lyn's light and life.

Randy Henderson – As a graduate of the United States Naval Academy, a former nuclear submarine officer, a well respected litigation attorney and a master mediator using his skill of dispute resolution, Randy knows the importance of the art of communication and finding the good in life. He is a father, grandfather, peak performance coach, and a true model for those seeking to live a life of integrity, success and meaning.

Roxana Hetzel – Originally from Philly, Roxana now lives in Manhattan Beach, California with her husband and two crazy dogs. She is an aficionado of Muay Thai kickboxing, live music, and world travel. As part of a large extended family, Roxana looks forward to making her own family grow very soon!

Margaret Irving – "Chili" is the embodiment of commitment, love, passion, contribution, AND ENERGY! Hence, her moniker, "The Energy Rocket." She is a world champion power lifter and international coach on business, presentation skills, content creation and delivery. She shares how to get the Energy Edge through rebound exercise. Chili is also an event manager, and serves as one of Tony Robbins' main room managers globally and lives to fulfill her mission, "To inspire others to raise their energy level so they can fulfill their life's dreams."

Chuck Hogan – Chuck is a devoted husband, father, friend and highly successful entrepreneur. He lives his life in Dallas and is humbled and honored by his parent's love that provided him with a life filled with multicultural diversity and life lessons. He serves others as a trainer for a personal development company helping people to experience their magical moments and life with grace, love and gratitude.

Ashton Kloes – Swim team, painter, skier, and beach boy, Ashton lives his life with appreciation for the full sensory experience of life. He enjoys and appreciates all he can see, hear, touch, smell and especially taste – as he is a cook who enjoys posting pictures of his creations for the world to enjoy. He and his father share a love of the ocean and are at their best in the waves.

Cristian Kloes – Club volleyball, artist, snowboarder, and surfer, Cristian plays full out in all he does, whether it's being a star student or a role model big brother. His intense focus on life will drive him to the future of his dreams.

Gregory Kloes – Greg is a historian and master instructor in European History. When he isn't immersed in what Napoleon or King Henry the 8th were thinking centuries ago, he surfs the waves in Manhattan Beach and around the world, grateful for the gifts of the ocean and the power of this earth.

Felix, Sam, Emma & Max Lin – The Lin Family are diehard Los Angeles Kings hockey fans and live their passion as a family through enjoying the magical moments in every game and showing their children what it means to dedicate themselves to whatever passion inspires them.

Woody Marks – Outrageous would be a mild word for Woody. He lives every moment in a powerfully inspired state growing his multi-city businesses in Alabama and Louisiana. He spends a huge amount of time serving others through his humor, intensity and dedication to the greater good.

Oliver Mausner – From the time he was young, Oliver set his intention, focus, and commitment to his various passions including playing college basketball. He is now a shooting guard at Claremont McKenna College, studies psychology and will pursue a career in sports. He is a role model for the phrase, "where focus goes, energy flows." Also known as DJ Omas, Oliver shares his love of music through his passion as a DJ.

Samantha Mausner – An eye for life and a zest for living, Sammy is an inspired photographer capturing life's magical moments through the lens of her camera. Sammy's independence and natural social skills will carry her into the future of her dreams. She exhibits her social consciousness through her varied work at homeless shelters, orphanages and other places in need.

Dave, Dawn & Henry Neilson – The Neilson family embodies the international flavor of England, New Zealand and America. Their love of magical moments comes from four-year old Henry who holds his parents accountable each night at dinner when he reminds them to share the magic in their lives. They are a family who embodies elegance, gratitude and an immense love for each other and those closest to them.

Nick Palmer – Surfing waves around the world, basketball, and beach volleyball – athletics at its best…Focus, dedication, commitment, a career at its finest…Love, wisdom, serving – contribution to family, friends and the greater good at its most inspirational…Welcome to Nick.

Carolyn Sampson – Based in Colorado Springs, Carolyn is a woman who walks her talk with love, energy and strength. A business expert, a trainer for a personal development company, a shining light in her spiritual community and so much more, she lives each day knowing that God serves through her spirit and guides her to inspiring others leading them to their own greatness.

Kevin Sousa – Kevin is an avid waterman, artist and musician, a PhD candidate in Depth Psychotherapy and is a highly respected Marriage and Family Therapist. He lives to appreciate and recognize the gifts of life; how they appear through people, places and things as symbols that guide all of us. He is an inspiring role model as an environmental and community activist in his home of Hermosa Beach, CA where he lives with his wife Patti and dog Jaxon.

Patti Sousa – Patti is a wise and dedicated example of what it means to stand up for what is right and good in this world. She is the Chief of Staff for IT Finance at Voya Financial and also takes action in her community by working tirelessly to protect the environment. She is true blue in her love of her husband Kevin, family, friends, and in her devotion to caring for our four-legged friends, especially her dog Jaxon.

Stacy Stevens – Stacy is a role model for caring deeply about what's important in life, especially family. She raised two boys to live their dreams of playing Division One college hockey. She is dedicated to rescuing our less fortunate four-legged furry friends and finding them loving homes.

Tammy Tantilla – Tammy is an impactful and effective personal life coach helping couples and individuals create the passion and love absolutely necessary to manifest the relationship and life that dreams are made of. Based in Chicago, she and her husband Mike live and breath love for each other raising the standards of everyone they touch.

Kelly Thormodsgaard – A resident of Manhattan Beach, California, there are many who refer to Kelly as a spiritual angel. As a beautiful and devoted wife, mother, teacher and friend, her guiding light and her intentions are powerful and continue to manifest answers to prayers like no other. Her feminine essence and true devotion to God captivate those who know and love her.